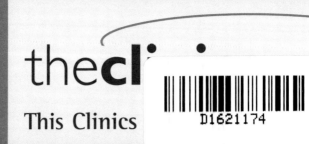

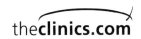
theclinics.com

SURGICAL ONCOLOGY CLINICS OF NORTH AMERICA

The Evolution of Radical Cancer Surgery

GUEST EDITOR
Marvin J. Lopez, MD

CONSULTING EDITOR
Nicholas J. Petrelli, MD

July 2005 • Volume 14 • Number 3

SAUNDERS

An Imprint of Elsevier, Inc.
PHILADELPHIA   LONDON   TORONTO   MONTREAL   SYDNEY   TOKYO

W.B. SAUNDERS COMPANY
A Division of Elsevier Inc.

1600 John F. Kennedy Boulevard, Suite 1800 • Philadelphia, PA 19103-2899

http://www.theclinics.com

SURGICAL ONCOLOGY CLINICS   Volume 14, Number 3
OF NORTH AMERICA   ISSN 1055-3207
July 2005   ISBN 1-4160-2789-0
Editor: Catherine Bewick

The ideas and opinions expressed in the *Surgical Oncology Clinics of North America* do not necessarily reflect those of the Publisher. The Publisher does not assume any responsibility for any injury and/or damage to persons or property arising out of or related to any use of the material contained in this periodical. The reader is advised to check the appropriate medical literature and the product information currently provided by the manufacturer of each drug to be administered to verify the dosage, the method and duration of administration, or contra-indications. It is the responsibility of the treating physician or other health care professional, relying on independent experience and knowledge of the patient, to determine drug dosages and the best treatment for the patient. Mention of any product in this issue should not be construed as endorsement by the contributors, editors, or the Publisher of the product or manufacturers' claims.

Surgical Oncology Clinics of North America (ISSN 1055-3207) is published quarterly by W.B. Saunders Company. Corporate and editorial offices: 1600 John F. Kennedy Boulevard, Suite 1800, Philadelphia, PA 19103-2899. Accounting and circulation offices: 6277 Sea Harbor Drive, Orlando, FL 32887–4800. Periodicals postage paid at Orlando, FL 32862, and additional mailing offices. Subscription prices are $165.00 per year (US individuals), $244.00 (US institutions) $83.00 (US student/resident), $188.00 (Canadian individuals), $295.00 (Canadian institutions), $113.00 (Canadian student/resident), $225.00 (foreign individuals), and $295.00 (foreign institutions) $113.00 (foreign student/resident). Foreign air speed delivery is included in all *Clinics* subscription prices. All prices are subject to change without notice. POST-MASTER: Send address changes to *Primary Care: Clinics in Office Practice*, W.B. Saunders Company. Periodicals Fulfillment. Orlando, FL 32887–4800. **Customer Service: 1-800-654-2452 (US). From outside the United States, call 1-407-345-4000. E-mail: hhspcs@wbsaunders.com.**

Reprints. For copies of 100 or more, of articles in this publication, please contact the Commercial Reprints Department, Elsevier Inc., 360 Park Avenue South, New York, New York 10010-1710. Tel. (212) 633-3813 Fax: (212) 462-1935 email: reprints@elsevier.com.

Surgical Oncology Clinics of North America is covered in *Index Medicus and EMBASE/Excerpta Medica, Current Contents/Clinical Medicine, and ISI/BIOMED.*

Printed in the United States of America.

CONSULTING EDITOR

NICHOLAS J. PETRELLI, MD, MBNA Endowed Medical Director, Helen F. Graham
Cancer Center, Newark, Delaware; and Professor of Surgery, Thomas Jefferson
University, Philadelphia, Pennsylvania

GUEST EDITOR

MARVIN J. LOPEZ, MD, Professor of Surgery, Tufts University School of Medicine;
Vice-Chairman, Department of Surgery, and Chief, General and Oncologic Surgery,
Caritas St. Elizabeth's Medical Center of Boston, Boston, Massachusetts

CONTRIBUTORS

STANLEY W. ASHLEY, MD, Frank Sawyer Professor of Surgery, Harvard Medical School;
Vice-Chairman of Surgery, Department of Surgery, Brigham and Women's Hospital,
Boston, Massachusetts

LIMARIS BARRIOS, MD, Clinical Associate, Surgery, Tufts University School of
Medicine; Department of Surgery, Caritas St. Elizabeth's Medical Center of Boston,
Boston, Massachusetts

BLAKE CADY, MD, FACS, Professor of Surgery, Brown Medical School; Rhode Island
Hospital, Department of Surgery, Providence, Rhode Island

DAVID B. CHESSIN, MD, Clinical Research Fellow, Colorectal Service, Department of
Surgery, Memorial Sloan-Kettering Cancer Center, New York, New York

THOMAS E. CLANCY, MD, Instructor in Surgery, Harvard Medical School; Associate
Surgeon, Department of Surgery, Brigham and Women's Hospital, Boston,
Massachusetts

MICHAEL R. DiSIENA, DO, Surgical Oncology Fellow, Department of Surgery, Roger
Williams Medical Center, Providence, Rhode Island

JENNE E. GARRETT, MD, Division of Urology, University of Kentucky Chandler Medical
Center, Lexington, Kentucky

JOSE G. GUILLEM, MD, MPH, Associate Attending Surgeon, Colorectal Service,
Department of Surgery, Memorial Sloan-Kettering Cancer Center; Associate Professor
of Surgery, Cornell University Medical College, New York, New York

SARAH H. HUGHES, MD, Division of Gynecologic Oncology, St. Elizabeth's Medical
Center of Boston; Tufts University School of Medicine, Boston, Massachusetts

LARRY R. KAISER, MD, The John Rhea Barton Professor and Chairman, Department of Surgery, University of Pennsylvania School of Medicine, Philadelphia, Pennsylvania

JOHN M. KANE III, MD, Department of Surgical Oncology–Melanoma/Sarcoma, Roswell Park Cancer Institute; Assistant Professor of Surgery, State University of New York at Buffalo, Buffalo, New York

WILLIAM G. KRAYBILL, MD, Department of Surgical Oncology–Chief Melanoma/Sarcoma, Roswell Park Cancer Institute; Professor of Surgery, State University of New York at Buffalo, Buffalo, New York

JOHN C. KUCHARCZUK, MD, Assistant Professor of Surgery, Section of Thoracic Surgery, University of Pennsylvania School of Medicine, Philadelphia, Pennsylvania

WALTER LAWRENCE, Jr, MD, Professor of Surgery Emeritus, Medical College of Virginia, Richmond, Virginia

MARVIN J. LOPEZ, MD, Professor of Surgery, Tufts University School of Medicine; Vice-Chairman, Department of Surgery, and Chief, General and Oncologic Surgery, Caritas St. Elizabeth's Medical Center of Boston, Boston, Massachusetts

SUBRAMANIAN NATARAJAN, FRCS, Fellow, Department of Surgery, Roger Williams Medical Center, Providence, Rhode Island

KEPAL N. PATEL, MD, Head and Neck Service, Memorial Sloan-Kettering Cancer Center, New York, New York

RANDALL G. ROWLAND, MD, PhD, Division of Urology, University of Kentucky Chandler Medical Center, Lexington, Kentucky

JATIN P. SHAH, MD, FACS, Hon. FRCS (Edin), Hon. FRACS, Hon. FDSRCS (Lond), Head and Neck Service, Memorial Sloan-Kettering Cancer Center, New York, New York

MICHAEL A. STELLER, MD, Clinical Professor of Obstetrics and Gynecology, Tufts University School of Medicine; Director, Division of Gynecologic Oncology, St. Elizabeth's Medical Center of Boston, Boston, Massachusetts

CHARU TANEJA, MD, FACS, Clinical Assistant Professor, Department of Surgery, Boston University School of Medicine, Boston, Massachusetts; Surgical Oncologist, Department of Surgery, Roger Williams Medical Center, Providence, Rhode Island

LUCRECIA TRABANINO, MD, Tufts University School of Medicine; Department of Surgery, Caritas St. Elizabeth's Medical Center of Boston, Boston, Massachusetts

HAROLD J. WANEBO, MD, Professor of Surgery, Department of Surgery, Boston University School of Medicine, Boston, Massachusetts; Adjunct Professor of Surgery, Department of Surgery, Brown University School of Medicine; Chief, Division of Surgical Oncology, Department of Surgery, Roger Williams Medical Center, Providence, Rhode Island

DAVID P. WINCHESTER, MD, FACS, Department of Surgery, Evanston Northwestern Healthcare, Evanston, Illinois; Department of Surgery, Northwestern University Medical School, Chicago, Illinois

CONTENTS

These factors have prompted practicing surgeons to adopt a more cautionary and conservative approach in the oncologic management of gastric cancer.

Popularized by Whipple and others in the first half of the twentieth century, pancreaticoduodenectomy today is the most common procedure performed for periampullary and pancreatic neoplasms. The technical and physiologic challenges posed by this procedure have resulted until recently in considerable perioperative mortality. With advances in surgical care and standardization of technique, mortality of less than 5% is now common, in experienced hands. This article reviews the history of pancreatic resection for treating cancer, the refinement of the procedure over subsequent decades, controversies in technique, and the current status of pancreaticoduodenectomy.

This article reviews the history of radical procedures for each urologic organ. Examples from the nineteenth century to the present are explored. Emphasis is placed on the evolution and current status of radical surgical procedures for treating renal, adrenal, bladder, prostatic, penile, and testicular cancers.

Abdominoperineal resection (APR) has been used for almost a century in the surgical management of rectal cancer. The evolution of this procedure over time parallels advances in the surgical management of cancer and provides an interesting perspective on the management of this disease. Our aim is to provide an historic perspective on the development of the APR and review the current issues and indications related to this procedure.

This article discusses the surgical results of pelvic exenteration for primary and recurrent rectosigmoid adenocarcinomas. This cancer site represents the most common clinical scenario and area of interest for general surgeons, surgical oncologists, and colorectal surgeons. Discussion includes the indications for surgery and preoperative evaluation, technique modifications, morbidity, mortality, and survival.

FORTHCOMING ISSUES

RECENT ISSUES

THE CLINICS ARE NOW ONLINE!

Access your subscription at:
http://www.theclinics.com

ELSEVIER
SAUNDERS

Surg Oncol Clin N Am
14 (2005) xi–xii

SURGICAL
ONCOLOGY CLINICS
OF NORTH AMERICA

Foreword

The Evolution of Radical Cancer Surgery

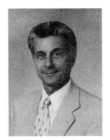

Nicholas J. Petrelli, MD
Consulting Editor

This issue of the *Surgical Oncology Clinics of North America* has as its Guest Editor Marvin J. Lopez, MD. I can't think of a more experienced individual to be the Guest Editor for an issue entitled "The Evolution of Radical Cancer Surgery." Dr. Lopez' experience in this area of oncology is recognized internationally. Just as importantly, he has successfully invited senior authors chosen particularly for their recognized experience in their respective fields of surgical oncology. Each of the authors in this issue presents a historical perspective of radical surgery in the past and in its current role, both alone and as part of the multidisciplinary team approach to many of the solid tumors discussed.

The theme of this issue is best described by Dr. Lopez in his preface when he states that "We must prepare future generations of surgeons to recognize the importance of obtaining cancer-free surgical resection margins and adequate lymphadenectomy, while avoiding violating or rupturing cancer-bearing organs and disrupting regional lymphatics in close proximity to the target organ." This type of experience along with the knowledge of the role of the radiation and medical oncologist is what separates the surgical oncologist from the general surgeon.

Surgical oncology fellows and residents will benefit tremendously from this issue. Radical surgery in head and neck, pancreatic, and gastric cancer are only a few of the topics described in this issue. Of course, the article on pelvic exenteration written by Dr. Lopez is outstanding and is a must-read for residents and fellows.

I congratulate Dr. Lopez and his colleagues for an outstanding issue of the *Surgical Oncology Clinics of North America.* I would also like to congratulate Dr. Lopez for finalizing this issue far earlier than the original time line. As my colleagues know, it is highly unusual for surgeons to complete articles ahead of schedule. It demonstrates that experienced and highly motivated individuals can accomplish anything that they want.

Nicholas J. Petrelli, MD
Helen F. Graham Cancer Center
4701 Ogletown-Stanton Road, Suite 1213
Newark, DE 19713, USA
Department of Surgery
Thomas Jefferson University
College Building, 1025 Walnut Street
Philadelphia, PA 19107, USA

E-mail address: npetrelli@christianacare.org

ELSEVIER
SAUNDERS

Surg Oncol Clin N Am
14 (2005) xiii–xv

SURGICAL
ONCOLOGY CLINICS
OF NORTH AMERICA

Preface

The Evolution of Radical Cancer Surgery

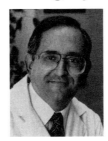

Marvin J. Lopez, MD
Guest Editor

In the last 150 years, the evolution of cancer surgery has been nothing short of spectacular. A close look at the mid–eighteenth century surgical panorama reveals a fascinating era of observation and discovery. Among these are observations on the natural history of malignant neoplasms usually diagnosed at late clinical stages. Primitive attempts at eradicating these tumors resulted in unacceptable human suffering and mortality. Toward the end of the eighteenth century, the clinico-pathologic features of malignant disease were so accurately described that they formed the basis for modern surgery and medicine. Even so, few medical conditions—and only rarely malignancy—could be cured by the likes of nineteenth century pioneers such as Billroth and Osler.

Advances in anatomic and clinical pathology, antisepsis, and anesthesia in the mid-1800s made it possible at the end of the nineteenth century and into the first 50 years of the twentieth century for European and American surgeons to develop radical operations for the cure of cancer. Radical surgery was developed out of the necessity to eradicate locally advanced malignant neoplasms that at the time of diagnosis had involved adjacent tissues and organs or regional lymph nodes. Further advances in antimicrobial therapy,

doi:10.1016/j.soc.2005.05.007   *surgonc.theclinics.com*

blood transfusion, nutritional support, and refinements in surgical technique reduced the morbidity and mortality of these operations to acceptable levels, such that the concept of an en bloc dissection has been from the early twentieth century onward an anatomically sound surgical approach.

During the last four decades, the surgical treatment of malignant tumors has been modified by the emergence of effective chemotherapeutic agents, improvement in radiation therapy technology and diagnostic imaging, prospectively randomized clinical trials, and early cancer detection practices. Further appreciation of tumor biology as a determinant of prognosis, quality of life issues, evidence-based medicine and increasing participation in clinical protocols are among the factors that have changed, for the better, the manner in which surgical oncology is practiced. It is an undisputed fact that more conservative resections, particularly when associated with effective adjuvant therapy, can improve quality of life in cancer patients without compromising cure. The success of the more conservative approach has spawned a trend to cast a negative connotation onto the concept of radical resection. This perception, when taken to the extreme, can result in neglect or trivialization of cancer operations and catastrophe for the patient. One needs to bear in mind that a good oncologic resection alone is responsible for the cure of the majority of cancers.

Even in the current era of multimodal treatment of cancer, those of us bearing responsibility for teaching must prepare future generations of surgeons to recognize the importance of obtaining cancer-free surgical resection margins and adequate lymphadenectomy, while avoiding violating or rupturing cancer-bearing organs and disrupting regional lymphatics in close proximity to the target organ. Knowledge and consistent application of these concepts, along with experience integrating radiation and chemotherapy in the pre- or postoperative treatment strategy, is what defines the modern surgical oncologist.

The general theme of this issue of the *Surgical Oncology Clinics of North America* is the evolution of cancer surgery. Each article takes a historical perspective toward the past and current role of radical surgery for the majority of cancers, where surgery retains a prominent role. The contributing senior authors were chosen for their recognized experience in their respective fields. The result is an issue that provides the reader not with an encyclopedic historical review but with an authoritative overview of an operation for cancer that still has a major role, perhaps modified to conform to the current standards of multimodal treatment of cancer. I am indebted to these authors for their excellent work and am privileged to have organized this issue, which will be referenced for many years. I also am indebted to my editorial assistant, Sarah Boardman, for her work in preparing and revising the manuscripts for this issue.

Marvin J. Lopez, MD
Tufts University School of Medicine
Caritas St. Elizabeth's Medical Center of Boston
736 Cambridge Street
Boston, MA 02135, USA

E-mail address: Marvin.Lopez.MD@caritaschristi.org

ELSEVIER
SAUNDERS

Surg Oncol Clin N Am
14 (2005) 441–446

SURGICAL
ONCOLOGY CLINICS
OF NORTH AMERICA

Radical Surgery for Cancer:
A Historical Perspective

Walter Lawrence Jr, MD[a], Marvin J. Lopez, MD[b,c,*]

[a]Medical College of Virginia, Richmond, VA 23298, USA
[b]Tufts University School of Medicine, 136 Harrison Avenue, Boston, MA 02111, USA
[c]Department of Surgery, Caritas St. Elizabeth's Medical Center of Boston,
736 Cambridge Street, Boston, MA 02135, USA

The distinguished contributors to this volume describe in detail the development and refinement of "radical" operations for cancer of specific anatomic sites. They have done so as true authorities in their respective fields, and many of them play a major role in recent medical history. However, as two surgeons who have had the privilege and pleasure of living and working through this changing era, particularly since the 1940s (WL) and the 1970s (MJL), with a combined clinical experience of over 80 years since graduating from medical school, we decided to add this philosophic commentary on the history of the evolution of some of these concepts over the time we have been involved. We both learned and worked with a number of pioneers of "cancer surgery," both past and present. These observations have led us to offer this perspective.

In the mid 1800s, after the development of general anesthesia, surgery for cancer became much more feasible than it had been earlier. Working in the patient's home, Ephraim McDowell removed a massive ovarian tumor, as early as 1809, but it was not until the latter half of the nineteenth century that cancer surgery really developed. Halsted (radical mastectomy), Billroth (gastrectomy, laryngectomy, hemipelvectomy, and prostatectomy), Weir, von Mikulicz, and Charles Mayo (colon cancer), Kocher at the turn of the century, and Lahey in the first quarter of the twentieth century (thyroid), George Crile and Nicholas Senn, Roswell Park, and Hayes Martin (head and neck cancer), and Clark and Wertheim (uterine cancer) all developed or refined operations for cancers of these sites. During the first 40 years of the twentieth century, new procedures for other cancers were developed by

* Corresponding author. Department of Surgery, Caritas St. Elizabeth's Medical Center of Boston, 736 Cambridge Street, Boston, MA 02135.
    E-mail address: Marvin.Lopez.MD@caritaschristi.org (M.J. Lopez).

1055-3207/05/$ - see front matter © 2005 Elsevier Inc. All rights reserved.
doi:10.1016/j.soc.2005.05.003   surgonc.theclinics.com

Miles (abdominoperineal resection in 1908), Graham (pneumonectomy in 1933), Whipple (pancreaticoduodenectomy in 1935), and Brunschwig (pelvic exenteration in 1948). With few exceptions, all of these operations focused only on the feasibility of removing the part of the anatomical structure containing the cancer. The additional principle of also excising the regional lymph nodes en bloc, first advanced by Halsted, also was emphasized by Miles for rectal cancer and by Crile for head and neck cancer. In contrast to some operations developed later, all of these procedures were established on the basis of either "armchair logic" or limited retrospective clinicopathologic studies. These were purely empirical developments. The surgical pioneers of the late 1800s and early 1900s reacted with surgical therapies designed to control locally advanced disease that was invariably present at the time of diagnosis. The era of early cancer detection practices, especially for breast and cervical carcinomas, would change to a dramatic extent the surgical philosophies in the mid twentieth century.

This commentary focuses on the period from the 1940s to the present. Concurrent events such as improvements in anesthesia and blood transfusion and the development of antimicrobials made a real extension of operative surgery feasible at this time. Looking back on the expansion of operations for cancer that occurred after World War II, it is clear that Dr. Halsted's concepts for the treatment of breast cancer were those that came into use for the treatment of many cancers. He had stressed the importance of removing the entire organ from which the cancer had originated (in his case, the breast). He also stressed en bloc resection of regional lymphatics in continuity with the primary lesion. These ideas were challenged and at least partially disproved by later clinical trials of the National Surgical Adjuvant Breast Project (NSABP) led by Bernard Fisher, but they were the true basis for a real extension of the operations for cancer beginning in the late 1940s. In addition, retrospective clinicopathologic studies of the various cancers were used as additional supporting evidence for the total or subtotal removal of various organs, extending the limits of regional lymph node dissection to include lymph nodes farther away than regional nodes, and the inclusion of additional organs invaded by or adherent to the cancer. These were the years of the concept "the bigger the operation, the bigger chance for cure!" For example, in 1950, Owen Wagensteen, one of the great American surgeons of the twentieth century, proposed that Halsted's radical mastectomy was obsolete and that the attack on breast cancer should include both internal mammary lymph node chains along with mediastinal and supraclavicular neck dissection.

A number of such operative extensions were initiated in the late 1940s, and subsequently, Dr. Brunschwig of the University of Chicago and, later, the Memorial Sloan-Kettering Cancer Center (MSKCC) performed many radical resections for gastrointestinal cancer. He also performed his first total pelvic exenteration for recurrent cervical cancer in 1946 when one of the authors (WL) was a student on his general surgical service. Dr. Eugene

Bricker (MJL's mentor) not only performed similar operations in the early 1940s but also initiated and perfected the very important ileal conduit for urinary diversion, as well. He later reported novel surgical approaches for pelvic reconstruction in cases of gastrointestinal and genitourinary fistulas resulting from extensive pelvic irradiation.

In breast surgery, total excision of the breast with both pectoral muscles and regional lymph node dissection (radical mastectomy) had been in vogue a long time, but Jerome Urban convinced one of us (WL) that by expanding the nodal excision to include the internal mammary lymph nodes along with a disk of chest wall was a vital treatment improvement. Everett Sugarbaker of Columbia, Missouri (one of MJL's predecessors at the Ellis Fischel Cancer Center) described a similar operation using an identical philosophy (eg, increasing the extent of nodal excision increases cure rates). Interestingly, recent data suggest that the number of lymph nodes excised during colectomy for colon cancer appears to have a prognostic significance. Lahey, Longmire, Pack, and McNeer all applied the concept of total removal of the organ involved and extended lymph node dissection to the management of gastric cancer. Japanese surgeons adopted this philosophy after World War II, and their practice of radical lymphadenectomies are still in vogue. One of us (WL), as a Fellow in training at MSKCC was actually the coauthor of a paper describing a "more thorough operation for gastric cancer" in 1951, despite the fact that he personally participated only in the pathologic studies at that time. Parenthetically, McNeer and one of us (WL) reported an analysis a decade later that argued against the value of this wider resection in favor of a more extended lymph node dissection. However, scientific data that proved this point awaited the superb randomized clinical trial of extended lymph node dissection from the Dutch trial, first reported in 1999. Meanwhile, to obtain an improved surgical resection margin and aim at what is today referred to as an R0 resection, one of us (MJL) extended Bricker's and Brunschwig's approach to pelvic exenteration by incorporating involved portions of the bony pelvis in what is referred to as a composite pelvic exenteration, with reasonably good results. Thus, the favorable biology of certain neoplasms justifies a more extensive salvage operation, even in the twenty-first century.

Similar extensions of operative procedures for head and neck cancer were pioneered by Grant Ward of Johns Hopkins and Hayes Martin of MSKCC (both of whom were teachers for WL in the 1940s and 1950s). Expansion of the lymph node dissection for colorectal cancer and for cancer of the cervix occurred as well during this era. The major expansion of the scope of the actual operative procedures for cancer during these years is what made what we now call "surgical oncology" so appealing to many of us younger surgeons who had a strong interest in the operating room. With the evolution of changing paradigms in cancer care, both of the authors became associated with and contributed to the teaching of modern surgical oncology, emphasizing the biologic features of disease, rather than the dogmatic anatomic principles of resection.

Although the pendulum of dealing with the extent of surgery for cancer had clearly swung a little farther than we now believe reasonable, anyone questioning the status quo received some ridicule from many quarters in the 1950s and 1960s. George Crile Jr, of the Cleveland Clinic, questioned the value of the high-mortality risk, low-cure rate operation for pancreatico-duodenectomy and the basic wisdom of axillary lymph node dissection for breast cancer. He was considered a maverick by the majority of surgeons of the day. Bernard Fisher and his cooperative trial group then had the audacity to question Dr. Halsted's hypotheses, on which so many of these operations of this era were based. Dr. Fisher was subsequently instrumental in the initiation of clinical trials that ultimately supported most of his own views that incorporated biologic concepts that were developed in the laboratory. He later received widespread acknowledgment for his leadership in this area, but he received his share of argument from Urban and others (the extended surgery "club") in the 1950s and 1960s, because he was a minority voice in those days. In more recent decades, Blake Cady, who provides insights into the area of lymphadenectomy for cancer in this issue, also has argued in terms of some of the currently established surgical policies, particularly of lymph node dissection for cancer. His views, however, have been considered more courteously because our surgical establishment has become more sophisticated scientifically.

Radical or extended surgery now has receded gradually somewhat over the last several decades, and the word radical has achieved some negative connotations. At the same time, surgical treatment results are actually better now than they ever were, despite much room for additional improvement. To what can we attribute these recent trends?

1. Probably our most important reason for less extensive operations at this time, as well as better results, is the fact that we now have an earlier diagnosis of cancer than in those earlier years. The extensive operation for breast cancer might well have been based on an inaccurate hypothesis, but the usual stage of cancers at diagnosis in Halsted's time was so different from now. We "grew up" at the height of the radical surgical revolution and matured during the course of more conservative surgical approaches. In breast cancer, for example, one of us (MJL) saw only classic Halstedian radical mastectomy performed during his internship year, learned modified radical mastectomy during his residency, and performed one of the first lumpectomies for breast cancer under the clinical trial conditions of the NSABP as a resident, and today he performs 80% breast preservation procedures for breast cancer. Naturally, screening by mammography led to the detection of cancers that are so amenable to more limited operations and to better treatment results. The same observations presently apply to colorectal cancer as a result of colorectal screening and, hopefully, may apply to lung cancer if the current spiral CT screening trials prove favorable.

2. The maturation of clinical trials methodology and its use in oncology and the growing acceptance of "evidence-based medicine" also are important developments affecting the choice of operative procedure. We attribute the initiation of randomized clinical trials to James Lind, who, in the 1700s, proved the benefits of citrus juice in the prevention of scurvy. However, the scientific use of prospective randomized clinical trials for most of our human cancers was established only in recent decades. Many colleagues should receive credit for this development, but in the surgical oncology area, Bernard Fisher's name stands out as a leader with major impact. These trials are what have led to many of the current standards of care for most human cancers.

3. Another factor adding to current changing trends in the choice of operation is the appreciation of the importance of patient function and cosmesis, currently known as "quality of life." Many of our very radical operations for head and neck cancer in the 1940s and 1950s led many patients to become unhappy, dysfunctional recluses, particularly those who underwent total mandibulectomy as part of the excision (the so-called "Andy Gump" operation). Improved reconstructive procedures certainly assisted with this problem without actually requiring a reduction in the extent of the operation, but improved adjuvant radiation and chemo-radiation techniques have allowed less extensive operations in some instances. For breast cancer, the NSABP trials not only altered some of the previous treatment hypotheses they gave patients more user-friendly operations from the standpoint of body image (eg, segmental mastectomy) by using adjuvant therapies.

4. In some instances, the reduction in the extent of the operation for cancer has been achieved recently by the introduction of other clinical innovations. For example, various imaging staging techniques and laparoscopic procedures have allowed more precise patient selection for extended surgery and the avoidance of such surgery for patients who would clearly not benefit. New equipment developments such as endoluminal staplers and endorectal ultrasonography have allowed more frequent sphincter preservation in the surgical management of rectal cancer. More recently, sentinel lymph node mapping and biopsy have been used to select patients for lymphadenectomy rather than using routine elective lymph node dissection. This technique, initiated by Morton a decade ago, clearly has refined the management of regional lymph node metastases for melanoma and, more recently, for breast cancer. All of these factors have played some role in the recent changes in our operative approach to cancer; however, earlier diagnosis and our use of the scientific method in well-performed clinical trials are probably the most important ones.

It has been exciting for both of us to have been involved in surgical oncology during the last half of the twentieth and the beginning of the twenty-first century and to have seen the many changes in treatment approach that have occurred. It has been exciting, as well, to have had the opportunity to rub elbows with many of those responsible for the evolution of cancer surgery during these times. What is really clear to us from this experience is that surgery for cancer has not and will not stand still. Advances in diagnosis, patient selection for operative treatment, and the individual treatments themselves will continue to take place as time goes on. Improvements that have occurred and will continue to occur in the field of adjuvant therapy will certainly affect the operation itself, as has been seen already in breast and anorectal cancer, and these improvements look promising for other gastrointestinal malignancies, as well. Also, targeted therapies are now being assessed that may further change our strategies. The next 50 years should have more innovations than the last 50, now that surgeons have evidence-based medicine for their decision-making process.

ELSEVIER
SAUNDERS

Surg Oncol Clin N Am
14 (2005) 447–459

SURGICAL
ONCOLOGY CLINICS
OF NORTH AMERICA

Evolution of Lymphadenectomy in Surgical Oncology

Subramanian Natarajan, FRCS[a],
Charu Taneja, MD, FACS[a,b],
Blake Cady, MD, FACS[c,*]

[a]Department of Surgery, Roger Williams Medical Center, 825 Chalkstone Avenue, Providence, RI 02908, USA
[b]Department of Surgery, Boston University School of Medicine, 715 Albany Street, Boston, MA 02118, USA
[c]Brown Medical School, Rhode Island Hospital, Department of Surgery, 593 Eddy Street, APC 4, Providence, RI 02903, USA

Lymphadenectomy, as an integral part of the field of surgical oncology, dates back to the sixteenth century. Since then, it has gone through phases, from minimal to supraradical operations, and now back to a minimally invasive approach. In many ways, the type of surgery performed on the lymphatic system as part of a cancer operation has paralleled the development of surgical techniques, the progress of anesthesia, and, most importantly, our understanding of the role of the lymphatic system underlying the metastatic process with, recently, an increased understanding of the molecular events of the progress from metastatic cell dissemination to the development of clinical metastases.

Historic aspects

Historically, breast cancer was one of the earliest cancers where the importance of the lymphatic system in the metastatic process was recognized, and it continues to serve as the paradigm by which the role of the lymphatic system in cancer is described. Ambrose Pare (born 1510) was among the earliest surgeons to recognize that the axillary lymph "glands" may be involved in breast cancer, and one of his contemporaries, Michael Servetus (born 1509) suggested that the axillary nodes should be removed as

* Corresponding author.
E-mail address: bcady@usasurg.org (B. Cady).

1055-3207/05/$ - see front matter © 2005 Elsevier Inc. All rights reserved.
doi:10.1016/j.soc.2005.04.005
surgonc.theclinics.com

part of the operation on breast cancer [1]. These findings were largely ignored but again, in the seventeenth century, Henri Le Dran (born 1685) and Jean Petit (born 1674) advocated the removal of the axillary nodes in breast cancer. They further concluded that breast cancer was curable in its early stages, where there was a benefit to removal of the axillary nodes, but the involvement of the axillary nodes signaled a worsened prognosis. This was further emphasized by a Scottish surgeon, James Syme (born 1799), who felt that the axillary nodes should be evaluated as part of the operation for breast cancer, but stated that the results were always unsatisfactory when the glands were involved, no matter how carefully they were removed [2]. Charles Moore (born 1821) and Sir Joseph Lister (born 1827) advocated a more radical approach to breast cancer surgery, and proposed that the division of the pectoral muscles would allow for a better exposure of the axillary contents. This was also made possible by the introduction of antiseptic techniques, which ushered in the era of modern surgery.

The first formal recorded reference to the technique of axillary dissection came in Joseph Pancoast's (born 1805) *Treatise on Operative Surgery* in 1844 [3]. Simultaneously, Samuel D. Gross (born 1805) removed the axillary glands only if they were grossly involved [4], but his son, Samuel W. Gross (born 1837), advocated a much more radical approach including excision of the overlying skin [5]. William Halsted (born 1852) and Willie Meyer (born 1854) simultaneously published papers advocating the systematic removal of nodes in continuity with the primary cancer in 1894 [6,7]. These papers presented the technique of lymphadenectomy in breast cancer in an anatomically logical and exact manner, and dispersed the technique by publications widely through the surgical community. This emphasis on the lymph nodes was simultaneously being seen in other cancers as well. Moynihan, in the early 1900s, emphasized that the resection of regional nodes was necessary in the cure of the patient with rectal cancer. He stated that "the surgery of malignant disease is not the surgery of organs; it is the anatomy of the lymphatic system" [8].

The first published account of melanoma, ascribed to John Hunter in 1787, was a nodal metastasis. Melanoma was further described by Laennec (1806), William Norris (1820), Pemberton (1858), Hutchison (1886), and Tennent (1885). Although Fergusson (1857) was the first to describe the excision of nodal metastases from melanoma, Herbert Snow proposed elective groin dissection for melanoma in 1892 [9]. The details of regional nodal resection technique were first described by Basset, in 1912, and were further refined by Taussig (1940), Baronofsky (1948), and Woodhall (1953), among others [10]. Preoperative lymphography was performed by Spratt early in 1965 [10].The oily dye used would remain in the lymph nodes at the completion of a lymph node dissection so that an on table a radiograph could be taken to confirm that the lymphadenectomy was complete.

Sir Geoffrey Keynes first described the role of radiation therapy (RT) in local control of cancer in 1930, and Robert McWhirter (born 1904) in 1948 demonstrated that axillary RT was effective in locoregional control in breast cancer [11]. This first aroused the controversy regarding surgical resection versus radiotherapy for locoregional control and its relationship to survival.

Although William Halsted reported the removal of supraclavicular lymph nodes as part of breast cancer operations, it was William Handley, in 1927, who advocated a more radical approach routinely to the treatment of breast cancer by removing the internal mammary nodes as well. This was followed by Jerome Urban (1952) and Owen Wangensteen (1950), among others, who pioneered the "supraradical mastectomy" in which the dissection was carried into the neck or mediastinum [12]. Although Patey and Dyson, in 1948, reported equivalent results from modified radical mastectomy compared with supraradical mastectomy [13], it was not until the1970s that the surgical trend for breast cancer management was deliberately directed toward limited procedures after publication of early trials demonstrated equivalent results. Axillary dissection in many instances became confined to sampling of level 1 nodes.

During this period, surgical treatment for gastric cancer was also undergoing changes. Since the first gastrectomy performed by Theodor Billroth in 1881, it took more than 70 years for McNeer, Pack and Lawrence (1950) to advocate from their superior results for an extended lymphadenectomy accompanying total gastrectomy [14,15]. This was quickly followed by Japanese surgeons (Maruyama and others), who took the extent of lymphadenectomy for gastric cancer to a still more radical level by defining 16 regional nodal stations to be removed [16,17]. Despite western series highlighting, the increased morbidity and mortality of extensive lymphadenectomy, along with discouraging survival benefits [14,15,18–21], Japanese series consistently reported a survival advantage from these procedures, thereby justifying them, but they ignored the effect of dramatic stage shifting that occurred as a result of screening with far fewer nodal metastases.

Although Gould (1960) described "sentinel lymph node" in radical resection for parotid cancer [22], and Cabanas defined the "sentinel lymph node" in penile cancer in 1977 [23], it was Morton, in 1992, who described and popularized the technique of identifying the sentinel lymph node in cutaneous melanoma using blue dye [24]. Krag (1993) used a gamma probe after injecting technetium sulfur colloid in breast cancer to identify the axillary sentinel lymph node [25], and Giuliani [26] used blue dye to also localize the sentinel axillary node. These two authors popularized these techniques for breast cancer, but combining the two techniques became the most widely accepted approach.

Anatomy of the lymphatic system

The first accurate descriptive anatomy of the lymphatic system was made by Gasparo Aselli, in 1622, when he noted that in dissecting a well-fed dog the mesenteric lacteals were engorged and visible, and drained to the central mesenteric nodes [27]. Jean Pecquet, in 1653 (thoracic ducts), Olof Rudbeck, and Thomas Bartholin, in 1653 (the term "Lymphatics"), Sappey, in 1888 (cutaneous lymphatics), and Von Recklinghausen (endothelial lining of lymph capillaries) all contributed to the understanding of the anatomy of the lymphatic system [28]. Virchow (1860) was a proponent of the concept that lymph nodes served a barrier function (ie, a "filter") to the spread of cancer [29]. With the advent of lymphangiography using a radio opaque dye by Kinmoth (1952), Ludwig described five different patterns of afferent and efferent lymph node lymphatics, thus demonstrating that a "filter" function was probably not the only issue [30] in cancer cell dissemination, as he noted that some afferent lymph vessels bypass lymph nodes entirely.

Apart from the bone marrow and the central nervous system, all parts of the body are drained by the lymphatic system. The lymph capillaries form a network that is far more extensive than that of the blood capillaries. The lymphatic capillaries are lined by a single layer of endothelial cells without intercellular gaps in the resting state. There are anchoring filaments attached to the outside of the endothelial cells that appear to control the entry of lymph from the interstitium. When the pressure or volume of the interstitial lymph increases, the anchoring filaments pull apart the adjacent lymphatic endothelial cells creating gaps thus allowing fluid to flow into the lymphatic capillaries [31]. The collecting lymph vessels (lymphatics) contain valves every 2 to 3 mm, and become double or trilayered vessels. These lymph vessels coalesce to form larger lymphatics that anatomically run roughly parallel to veins to drain to regional lymph nodes.

A typical lymph node has a convex cortical surface through which afferent lymphatics enter. Beneath the cortex lies a marginal sinus that has a delicate reticulum that may trap particulate matter. From the marginal sinus, anastomosing medullary sinuses penetrate into the pulp of the node where the cords of cells are composed of lymphocytes. In the hilum of the lymph node, lymph channels coalesce to form the efferent lymphatic vessels that leave the node. Some lymph fluid returns to the venous circulation directly via the veins that drain the lymph node. The efferent lymphatic vessels coalesce into larger collecting lymphatics that ultimately empty into either the large thoracic duct on the left or a smaller right thoracic duct, both of which drain into large veins at the root of the neck.

Pathobiology of lymphatic spread

The lymphatic system has only four described functions. (1) It returns interstitial fluid to the systemic circulation; (2) it transports absorbed nutrients from the intestines to the vascular space via major lymphatic channels; (3) it exposes B and T lymphocytes in the lymph nodes to foreign antigens (chemical, bacterial,viral, parasitic); and (4) it produces humoral antibodies or cell-mediated cytotoxic responses from the respective B or T cell lymph node lymphocytes exposed to foreign antigens. Generally, the lymph node lymphocytes do not produce antibodies or elicit cytotoxic responses for the innate tumor antigens ("self" not "foreign"), but there are exceptions.

Lymph nodes are a much later evolutionary development of the lymphatic system to enable a more sophisticated immunologic system to deal with the hostile external environment of bacteria, viruses, and parasites by bringing collections of lymphocytes into the lymphatic stream. Lymph nodes are a porous organ (not a filter) that presents foreign antigens to the lymphocytes, which develop their immunologic "reading," and then produce the respective B and T cell immunologic functions. Foreign antigens then generally pass through the porous lymph node to prevent blockage and obstruction that otherwise might occur if the lymph nodes were strictly filters. Radiolabeled tumor cells injected into afferent lymphocytes rapidly transit lymph nodes and appear in the efferent lymph and thoracic duct. Thoracic duct drainage and selective elimination of lymphocytes, but with return of the lymph to the body, rapidly produces an immunologically incompetent host. A lymphocyte-depleted host resulting from eliminating the dynamically circulating lymphocytes that intermittently populate lymph nodes will accept organ transplants. This emphasizes the primary antigen recognition function of lymph nodes, and indicates the totally incidental role of lymph nodes in cancer, which, with some exceptions, are not foreign antigens and elicit few if any immunologic responses.

The perceived methods and mechanisms by which cancer spreads via the lymphatic system have in the past influenced how cancer is treated surgically. The earliest theory of cancer cell dissemination, first proposed by William Handley (born 1872) and popularized by William Halsted (born 1852), was a mechanistic, "lymphatic dominant" theory, where lymph nodes acted as filters or mechanical barriers to the spread of cancer cells. It was theorized that there were direct lymphatic pathways between the breast and the breast cancer and the liver, brain, and other distant organ metastic sites. According to this theory, lymphadenectomy, by ablating the lymphatic pathways through which cancer cells traveled and lymph nodes that trapped or filtered out the cells, would prevent their further spread. This theory was questioned as early as the 1900s by finding metastases in distant sites in the absence of regional nodal metastases [32]. In retrospect, this could be explained by the fact that some lymphatics do not drain into the lymph nodes but reached the systemic circulation directly. By demonstrating that removal of regional axillary lymph nodes did not decrease distant metastases or alter survival compared with radiating or observing them, Fisher [33] proposed a biologic theory that cancer was a "systemic disease from outset." Cancer cells escaped from the primary organ simultaneously through both the lymphatics and the blood stream to create distant metastases. Fisher and colleagues [33–35] proposed that there was a complex interaction between tumor and host and that the presence of involved regional lymph nodes was a marker of a relationship that permitted the development of distant metastases or acted as a marker of metastatic potential. However, as screening programs for breast cancer and gastric cancer were implemented in the United States, Europe, and Japan, it was apparent that "early" cancers had an excellent long-term survival, thus questioning the "systemic from outset" theory. The most recent biologic theory of cancer cell dissemination succeeding the earlier "lymphatic dominant" and later "systemic from origin" postulates is the "spectrum model" enunciated by Hellman [36], based on his reports and those of Tubiana and Koscielny [37]. It postulates that primary cancers exhibit a spectrum of biologic behavior; some patients ($\pm 20\%$) display no capacity to create distant clinical metastases despite larger size or even the presence of a few nodal metastases, while a smaller proportion ($\pm 10\%$) even at earliest presentation have a high rate of dissemination, distant metastases, and poor survival, and are therefore examples of "systemic from origin" biology. In the great majority of patients (67%–75%), the capacity of the primary cancer to disseminate is a function of duration and size. With increasing clonal evolution as cancers persist and grow, they display increasing virulence and metastatic potential. In this "spectrum model" lymph node metastases may or may not precede distant metastases, and the presence of nodal involvement is a predictor for, rather than an instigator of, distant disease. Recent studies regarding interstitial fluid pressure in the vicinity of cancer [38,39], molecular cellular receptors and their expression [40], cytokines [41], angiogenesis [42], and lymphangiogenesis [43], leads to the conclusion that clinical metastasis to the regional lymph nodes and distant sites is a complex multistep process that is neither efficient nor readily predictable.

More recently, the frequent presence of cancer cells in bone marrow aspirates in the absence of regional nodal metastases has even brought the spectrum theory into question [44]. Cancer cells have been demonstrated in the bone marrow in a wide variety of cancers [44–48]. However the mere presence of these cancer cells does not always correlate with standard prognostic features of the primary cancer, and instead may be related to certain genetic or cellular features, such as cell surface characteristics or vessel endothelial features as well as the "dose" of circulating tumor cells, which may predict if metastatic cells will be biologically active [49,50]. Further, it has been appreciated that cancer cells may remain dormant in a transplant host organ for years [51] and then be reactivated after transplantation and donor immunosuppression, as demonstrated in reports of donor organs with latent metastatic cells that produce cancers in transplant recipients many years later [52].

It has been recognized that multiple cellular events need to occur for the development of a clinical metastasis. These include the detachment of a malignant cell from the primary tumor, entry of the cell into the lymphatic or vascular space, cell attachment to the endothelium of the distal organ artery, implantation and penetration through that vessel wall, and pro-gressive growth in the distant site [53–55]. This may require an adequate "dose" of tumor cells to initiate or continue the process to achieve a clinical metastasis, as in animal models [50]. Angiogenesis seems critical to the development of metastases larger than 2 to 3 mm diameter [42] by enabling the growth of implanted cell clusters beyond the capacity of mere diffusion of nutrients to create progressive growth and a clinical metastasis. Metastatic cells also have organ specificity, and selected tumor cells injected into nude mice show patterns of organ lodgement and growth similar to that seen in humans with specific distant organ metastatic patterns [56]. The molecular and genetic mechanisms involved in the specificity and selectivity of metastatic organ sites are only now being understood, but particular cytokines have been demonstrated to block lymph node-specific cells in breast cancer models [57,58].

Clinical implications of lymphadencectomy

Breast cancer

Prospective randomized trials, which began in the 1960s, indicated no survival benefit from extended radical mastectomy with internal mammary node dissection compared with radical mastectomy [59,60], and subsequent trials stressed the equivalent survival comparing of modified radical mastectomy to radical mastectomy [60]. With regard to axillary lymphade-nectomy, a randomized trial comparing radical mastectomy, total mastectomy with RT, and total mastectomy alone found no difference in the rate of distant metastases and survival in clinically node negative breast cancer patients after 25 years [61]. Of note, only 20% of these clinically node-negative patients without axillary dissection developed later clinical nodal metastases, despite the fact that over 40% of cases were known to have nodal metastases from the rate in the radical mastectomy group, thus demonstrating that leaving behind axillary nodes with metastatic disease had no significant impact on the overall outcome of the disease, and indeed, in only one-half of cases would later develop clinical node recurrences.

Melanoma

The beneficial effect of removing clinically uninvolved regional lymph nodes has been examined by four randomized controlled trials [62–65]. The World Health Organization melanoma oncology group and the Intergroup Melanoma surgical program randomized patients to elective lymph node dissection or observation for clinically negative nodes and found no survival benefit for immediate resection after over 9 years of follow-up. There were small subgroups who, on retrospective subset analysis, appeared to have benefited from elective lymph node dissection (accepting the morbidity of the procedure), but the analysis was flawed and the subset criteria had no biologic rational [66,67]. After this, sentinel lymph node biopsy came into practice, and the chance of testing these artificial subgroups in a randomized trial was lost. Currently, two trials (Sunbelt Melanoma trial and Multicenter Selective Lymphadenectomy trial) are evaluating sentinel lymph node biopsy of high-risk groups to be followed by lymph node dissection if occult metastatic disease is found; no results are yet available [68]. In summary, there is no convincing evidence at present of a survival benefit of immediate regional nodal dissection.

Gastric cancer

The extent of lymphadenectomy in gastric cancer surgery continues to be a controversial issue. Four randomized trials have specifically addressed this issue, and none of them showed any survival advantage for an extended lymph node dissection compared with a limited dissection accompanying gastrectomy [20,69–71]. All four trials encountered significantly increased morbidity and increased operative mortality in patients undergoing extended lymphadenectomy. In addition, two of the trials demonstrated no survival benefit even for extended gastric resection for distal gastric cancers, consistent with other data demonstration that more extensive surgery is not beneficial in terms of survival [20,72]. Recently, Wu and colleagues [73] reported a randomized comparison of D_1 lymphadenectomy to D_3 lymphadenectomy in patients with adenocarcinoma of the stomach. The authors again noted that extended lymphadenectomy was associated with more complications with the impact on survival not addressed.

Sarcoma, thyroid cancer, carcinoid, and islet cell cancers

Sarcomas infrequently have regional nodal metastases ($\pm 5\%$) but frequently have lung metastases. Some of these pulmonary metastases from sarcoma are curable by pulmonary resection, suggesting that the circulating sarcoma cells have a reduced capacity to grow in other organs but a selective orientation for the lungs. In low-risk thyroid cancer, and carcinoid and islet cell cancers, regional nodal involvement is very common but not adversely related to survival. Thus, young patients with differentiated thyroid cancer have regional nodal metastases in up to 75% of patients, yet have a 99% long-term survival, indicating a selective pattern of nodal metastases without risk of other organ clinical metastases. Carcinoid and pancreatic islet cell cancers are defined as cancers by nodal or other metastases and have frequent nodal metastases, but these are not associated with a poor outcome, because apparently these nodal metastasis cells have little capacity to grow in other organs.

Sentinel lymph node biopsy

Sentinel lymph node biopsy has been studied extensively in breast cancer and melanoma, but the concept of a sentinel lymph node evaluation has been investigated in many other solid organ cancers. Initially, the concept of sentinel lymph node biopsy was designed to evaluate the stage of the disease before lymphadenectomy, eliminating the need for regional node resection if the sentinel nodes were negative. Krag [25], Morton and colleagues [24], and Giuliano and colleagues [26], and many subsequent authors all demonstrated that sentinel lymph node evaluation is feasible, and accurately predicts the regional nodal status, and could be readily applied in practice in melanoma and breast cancer [24,26]. The analysis of the few removed sentinel lymph nodes enabled pathologists to do multiple sections and a far more careful analysis of a few nodes, rather than a single section of the 16 nodes usually obtained from an axillary dissection. This detailed examination has sharply increased (by 20%–30%) the proportion of "positive" nodes. Intraoperative assessment of sentinel lymph nodes using touch imprints and routine immunohistochemical staining is used by some to enable an immediate therapeutic lymphadenectomy if the nodes were positive, thus sparing the patient from a second procedure. However, intraoperative assessment may have unacceptable rates of false negative results (36%–71%) [74,75]. The increased yield of small macrometastases and micrometastases from regional lymph nodes by use of multiple thin sections and immunohistochemistry had been well demonstrated even in the presentinel lymph node era [76–78], and led to the recommendation for the current careful pathological analysis of sentinel lymph nodes [79]. With the technique of sentinel lymph node biopsy and the pathologic analysis now relatively standardized, the more recent focus is on the clinical significance of "positive" sentinel nodes. The most recent 6th edition of the American Joint Committee on Cancer Staging Manual defines nodal metastases less than 0.2 mm in extent and detected by immunohistochemical only as N_0, indicating the uncertain prognostic implication of these minor cancer cell discoveries. Not all "positive" sentinel lymph nodes require a subsequent therapeutic lymphadenectomy because studies have shown no increased risk of regional nodal recurrence after observation only for patients with a positive sentinel lymph node [80]. This thesis forms the hypothesis of the current American College of Surgeons Oncology Group Z-11 trial, which randomizes sentinel node-positive breast cancer patients to observation only or axillary dissection.

Summary

Lymphadenectomy, as an integral part of cancer operations, has been recognized and accepted for many years. Accurately defining the anatomy and physiology of the lymphatic system helps surgeons understand the complex pathobiology of lymphatic spread of malignant neoplasms. The clinical implications of regional lymph nodal metastases has taken a varied course over the years. Convincingly, the lymph node metastatic status has proven to be a major prognostic indicator of survival after surgery of most epithelial cancers. Attempts to improve the outcome of cancer operations by radical super radical, or extended lymphadenectomy has not been successful in improving survival, but unfortunately, has created increased morbidity. Sentinel lymph node biopsy has evolved as the best method of determining the lymph node status of breast cancer and melanoma patients with minimal morbidity, but whether this technique is applicable to other organ cancers has yet to be proven.

The outcome in cancers is determined by the presence of systemic spread to produce distant vital organ clinical metastases, but not caused by the regional nodal metastases or regional recurrence, which are indicators, but not instigators of poor outcome. The improved outcome after surgery in recent years is largely related to the earlier stage of disease resulting from screening and to the improvements in adjuvant therapy, not to more extensive surgery of the primary cancer or the regional node metastases.

References

[1] Robinson JO. Treatment of breast cancer through the ages. Am J Surg 1986;151(3):317–33.
[2] Syme J. Principles of surgery. London: H Balliere; 1842.
[3] Pancoast J. Treatise on operative surgery. Philadelphia: Carey & Hart; 1844.
[4] Cooper WA. The history of radical mastectomy. Ann Med Hist 1941;3:36.
[5] Gross SW. An analysis of two hundred and seven cases of carcinoma of the breast. Med News 1887;51:613.
[6] Halsted WS. The results of the operations for the cure of cancer of the breast performed at the Johns Hopkins Hospital from June 1889 to January 1894. Johns Hopkins Hosp Rep 1895;4:297.
[7] Meyer W. An improved method of the radical operation for carcinoma of the breast. Med Rec 1894;46:746.
[8] Moynihan GA. The surgical treatment of cancer of the sigmoid flexure and rectum. Surg Gynecol Obstet 1908;6:463–6.
[9] Neuhaus SJ, Clark MA, Thomas JM. Dr. Herbert Lumley Snow, MD, MRCS (1847–1930): the original champion of elective lymph node dissection in melanoma. Ann Surg Oncol 2004;11(9):875–8.
[10] Spratt J. Groin dissection. J Surg Oncol 2000;73(4):243–62.
[11] McWhirter R. The value of simple mastectomy and radiotherapy in the treatment of cancer of the breast. Br J Radiol 1948;21:599.
[12] Halsted WS. Parasternal invasion of the thorax in breast cancer and its suppresion by the use of radium tubes as an operative precaution. Surg Gynecol Obstet 1927;45:721–82.
[13] Patey DH, Dyson WH. The prognosis of carcinoma of the breast in relation to the type of operation performed. Br J Cancer 1948;2:7–13.
[14] Lawrence W Jr, McNeer G, Ortega LG, et al. Early results of extended total gastrectomy for cancer. Cancer 1956;9(6):1153–9.
[15] McNeer NG, Lawrence W Jr, Ashley AB, et al. End results in the treatment of gastric cancer. Surgery 1958;43(6):879–96.
[16] Maruyama K, Okabayashi K, Kinoshita T. Progress in gastric cancer surgery in Japan and its limits of radicality. World J Surg 1987;11(4):418–25.
[17] Kajitani T. The general rules for the gastric cancer study in surgery and pathology. Part I. Clinical classification. Jpn J Surg 1981;11(2):127–39.
[18] Bonenkamp JJ, van de Velde CJ, Kampschoer GH, et al. Comparison of factors influencing the prognosis of Japanese, German, and Dutch gastric cancer patients. World J Surg 1993; 17(3):410–4 [discussion: 415].

[19] Degiuli M, Sasako M, Calgaro M, et al. Morbidity and mortality after D1 and D2 gastrectomy for cancer: interim analysis of the Italian Gastric Cancer Study Group (IGCSG) randomised surgical trial. Eur J Surg Oncol 2004;30(3):303–8.

[20] Cuschieri A, Weeden S, Fielding J, et al. Patient survival after D1 and D2 resections for gastric cancer: long-term results of the MRC randomized surgical trial. Surgical Co-operative Group. Br J Cancer 1999;79(9–10):1522–30.

[21] Dent DM, Madden MV, Price SK. Randomized comparison of R1 and R2 gastrectomy for gastric carcinoma. Br J Surg 1988;75(2):110–2.

[22] Gould EA, Winship T, Philbin PH, et al. Observations on a "sentinel node" in cancer of the parotid. Cancer 1960;13:77–8.

[23] Cabanas RM. An approach for the treatment of penile carcinoma. Cancer 1977;39(2): 456–66.

[24] Morton DL, Wen DR, Wong JH, et al. Technical details of intraoperative lymphatic mapping for early stage melanoma. Arch Surg 1992;127(4):392–9.

[25] Krag DN, Weaver DL, Alex JC, et al. Surgical resection and radiolocalization of the sentinel lymph node in breast cancer using a gamma probe. Surg Oncol 1993;2(6):335–9 [discussion: 340].

[26] Giuliano AE, Kirgan DM, Guenther JM, et al. Lymphatic mapping and sentinel lymphadenectomy for breast cancer. Ann Surg 1994;220(3):391–8 [discussion: 398–401].

[27] Aselli G. Lactibus sive lacteis venis. Milan: J B Bidellius; 1627.

[28] Sappey MPC. Traite d'anatomie descriptive. Paris: A Delahaye et E Lacrosnier; 1888.

[29] Virchow R. Zur Diagnose der Krebse im Unterleibe. Med Reform 1849;45:248.

[30] Ludwig J. On bypasses of the lymphatic system and their relations to lymphogenic cancer metastasis. Pathol Microbiol (Basel) 1962;25:329–34.

[31] Leak LV, Burke JF. Electron microscopic study of lymphatic capillaries in the removal of connective tissue fluids and particulate substances. Lymphology 1968;1(2):39–52.

[32] Tyzzer EE. Factors in the production and growth of tumor metastases. J Med Res 1913;28: 309.

[33] Fisher B, Fisher ER. Biologic aspects of cancer-cell spread. Proc Natl Cancer Conf 1964;5: 105–22.

[34] Fisher ER, Fisher B. Recent observations on concepts of metastasis. Arch Pathol 1967;83(4): 321–4.

[35] Fisher B, Fisher ER. The interrelationship of hematogenous and lymphatic tumor cell disemination: an experimental study. Rev Inst Nac Cancerol (Mex) 1966;19:576–81.

[36] Harris JR. Natural history of breast cancer. In: Harris JR, Morrow M, editors. Diseases of the breast. Philadelphia: Lippincott-Raven; 1996.

[37] Koscielny S, Tubiana M, Le MG, et al. Breast cancer: relationship between the size of the primary tumour and the probability of metastatic dissemination. Br J Cancer 1984;49(6): 709–15.

[38] Jain RK, Munn LL, Fukumura D. Dissecting tumour pathophysiology using intravital microscopy. Nat Rev Cancer 2002;2(4):266–76.

[39] Nathanson SD, Nelson L. Interstitial fluid pressure in breast cancer, benign breast conditions, and breast parenchyma. Ann Surg Oncol 1994;1(4):333–8.

[40] Stacker SA, Caesar C, Baldwin ME, et al. VEGF-D promotes the metastatic spread of tumor cells via the lymphatics. Nat Med 2001;7(2):186–91.

[41] Baggiolini M. Chemokines and leukocyte traffic. Nature 1998;392(6676):565–8.

[42] Folkman J. Role of angiogenesis in tumor growth and metastasis. Semin Oncol 2002;29(6 Suppl 16):15–8.

[43] Karpanen T, Egeblad M, Karkkainen MJ, et al. Vascular endothelial growth factor C promotes tumor lymphangiogenesis and intralymphatic tumor growth. Cancer Res 2001; 61(5):1786–90.

[44] Braun S, Pantel K, Muller P, et al. Cytokeratin-positive cells in the bone marrow and survival of patients with stage I, II, or III breast cancer. N Engl J Med 2000;342(8):525–33.

[45] Gebauer G, Fehm T, Merkle E, et al. Micrometastases in axillary lymph nodes and bone marrow of lymph node-negative breast cancer patients—prognostic relevance after 10 years. Anticancer Res 2003;23(5b):4319–24.

[46] Bonavina L, Soligo D, Quirici N, et al. Bone marrow-disseminated tumor cells in patients with carcinoma of the esophagus or cardia. Surgery 2001;129(1):15–22.

[47] O'Sullivan GC, Sheehan D, Clarke A, et al. Micrometastases in esophagogastric cancer: high detection rate in resected rib segments. Gastroenterology 1999;116(3):543–8.

[48] Gerber B, Krause A, Muller H, et al. Simultaneous immunohistochemical detection of tumor cells in lymph nodes and bone marrow aspirates in breast cancer and its correlation with other prognostic factors. J Clin Oncol 2001;19(4):960–71.

[49] Braun S, Schlimok G, Heumos I, et al. ErbB2 overexpression on occult metastatic cells in bone marrow predicts poor clinical outcome of stage I–III breast cancer patients. Cancer Res 2001;61(5):1890–5.

[50] Cristofanilli M, Budd GT, Ellis MJ, et al. Circulating tumor cells, disease progression, and survival in metastatic breast cancer. N Engl J Med 2004;351(8):781–91.

[51] Naumov GN, MacDonald IC, Weinmeister PM, et al. Persistence of solitary mammary carcinoma cells in a secondary site: a possible contributor to dormancy. Cancer Res 2002; 62(7):2162–8.

[52] MacKie RM, Reid R, Junor B. Fatal melanoma transferred in a donated kidney 16 years after melanoma surgery. N Engl J Med 2003;348(6):567–8.

[53] Chambers AF, Naumov GN, Varghese HJ, et al. Critical steps in hematogenous metastasis: an overview. Surg Oncol Clin N Am 2001;10(2):243–55 [vii.].

[54] Fidler IJ. Seed and soil revisited: contribution of the organ microenvironment to cancer metastasis. Surg Oncol Clin N Am 2001;10(2):257–69 [vii–viiii.].

[55] Irjala H, Alanen K, Grenman R, et al. Mannose receptor (MR) and common lymphatic endothelial and vascular endothelial receptor (CLEVER)-1 direct the binding of cancer cells to the lymph vessel endothelium. Cancer Res 2003;63(15):4671–6.

[56] Brodt P. Adhesion mechanisms in lymphatic metastasis. Cancer Metastasis Rev 1991;10(1): 23–32.

[57] Espana L, Fernandez Y, Rubio N, et al. Overexpression of Bcl-xL in human breast cancer cells enhances organ-selective lymph node metastasis. Breast Cancer Res Treat 2004;87(1): 33–44.

[58] LeBedis C, Chen K, Fallavollita L, et al. Peripheral lymph node stromal cells can promote growth and tumorigenicity of breast carcinoma cells through the release of IGF-I and EGF. Int J Cancer 2002;100(1):2–8.

[59] Lacour J, Bucalossi P, Cacers E, et al. Radical mastectomy versus radical mastectomy plus internal mammary dissection. Five-year results of an international cooperative study. Cancer 1976;37(1):206–14.

[60] Turner L, Swindell R, Bell WG, et al. Radical versus modified radical mastectomy for breast cancer. Ann R Coll Surg Engl 1981;63(4):239–43.

[61] Fisher B, Jong-Hyeon J, Stewart A, et al. Twenty-five year follow-up of a randomized trial comparing radical mastectomy, total mastectomy, and total mastectomy followed by irradiation. N Engl J Med 2002;347(8):567–75.

[62] Cascinelli N, Morabito A, Santinami M, et al. Immediate or delayed dissection of regional nodes in patients with melanoma of the trunk: a randomised trial. WHO Melanoma Programme. Lancet 1998;351(9105):793–6.

[63] Veronesi U, Adamus J, Bandiera DC, et al. Inefficacy of immediate node dissection in stage 1 melanoma of the limbs. N Engl J Med 1977;297(12):627–30.

[64] Veronesi U, Adamus J, Bandiera DC, et al. Stage I melanoma of the limbs. Immediate versus delayed node dissection. Tumori 1980;66(3):373–96.

[65] Veronesi U, Adamus J, Bandiera DC, et al. Delayed regional lymph node dissection in stage I melanoma of the skin of the lower extremities. Cancer 1982;49(11): 2420–30.

[66] Balch CM, Soong SJ, Bartolucci AA, et al. Efficacy of an elective regional lymph node dissection of 1 to 4 mm thick melanomas for patients 60 years of age and younger. Ann Surg 1996;224(3):255–63 [discussion: 263–6].
[67] Balch CM, Soong S, Ross MI, et al. Long-term results of a multi-institutional randomized trial comparing prognostic factors and surgical results for intermediate thickness melanomas (1.0 to 4.0 mm). Intergroup Melanoma Surgical Trial. Ann Surg Oncol 2000;7(2):87–97.
[68] Morton DL, Thompson JF, Essner R, et al. Validation of the accuracy of intraoperative lymphatic mapping and sentinel lymphadenectomy for early-stage melanoma: a multicenter trial. Multicenter Selective Lymphadenectomy Trial Group. Ann Surg 1999;230(4):453–63 [discussion: 463–5].
[69] Bonenkamp JJ, Hermans J, Sasako M, et al. Extended lymph-node dissection for gastric cancer. Dutch Gastric Cancer Group. N Engl J Med 1999;340(12):908–14.
[70] Maeta M, Yamashiro H, Saito H, et al. A prospective pilot study of extended (D3) and superextended para-aortic lymphadenectomy (D4) in patients with T3 or T4 gastric cancer managed by total gastrectomy. Surgery 1999;125(3):325–31.
[71] Robertson CS, Chung SC, Woods SD, et al. A prospective randomized trial comparing R1 subtotal gastrectomy with R3 total gastrectomy for antral cancer. Ann Surg 1994;220(2):176–82.
[72] Bozzetti F, Marubini E, Bonfanti G, et al. Total versus subtotal gastrectomy: surgical morbidity and mortality rates in a multicenter Italian randomized trial. The Italian Gastrointestinal Tumor Study Group. Ann Surg 1997;226(5):613–20.
[73] Wu CW, Hsiung CA, Lo SS, et al. Randomized clinical trial of morbidity after D1 and D3 surgery for gastric cancer. Br J Surg 2004;91(3):283–7.
[74] Gibbs JF, Huang PP, Zhang PJ, et al. Accuracy of pathologic techniques for the diagnosis of metastatic melanoma in sentinel lymph nodes. Ann Surg Oncol 1999;6(7):699–704.
[75] Van Diest PJ, Torrenga H, Borgstein PJ, et al. Reliability of intraoperative frozen section and imprint cytological investigation of sentinel lymph nodes in breast cancer. Histopathology 1999;35(1):14–8.
[76] Prognostic importance of occult axillary lymph node micrometastases from breast cancers. International (Ludwig) Breast Cancer Study Group. Lancet 1990;335(8705):1565–8.
[77] Dowlatshahi K, Fan M, Bloom KJ, et al. Occult metastases in the sentinel lymph nodes of patients with early stage breast carcinoma: a preliminary study. Cancer 1999;86(6):990–6.
[78] Fisher ER, Swamidoss S, Lee CH, et al. Detection and significance of occult axillary node metastases in patients with invasive breast cancer. Cancer 1978;42(4):2025–31.
[79] Cibull ML. Handling sentinel lymph node biopsy specimens. A work in progress. Arch Pathol Lab Med 1999;123(7):620–1.
[80] Naik AM, Fey J, Gemignani M, et al. The risk of axillary relapse after sentinel lymph node biopsy for breast cancer is comparable with that of axillary lymph node dissection: a follow-up study of 4008 procedures. Ann Surg 2004;240(3):462–8 [discussion: 468–71].

ELSEVIER
SAUNDERS

Surg Oncol Clin N Am
14 (2005) 461–477

SURGICAL
ONCOLOGY CLINICS
OF NORTH AMERICA

Neck Dissection: Past, Present, Future

Kepal N. Patel, MD, Jatin P. Shah, MD, FACS,
Hon. FRCS (Edin), Hon. FRACS,
Hon. FDSRCS (Lond)*

*Head and Neck Service, Memorial Sloan–Kettering Cancer Center,
1275 York Avenue, New York, NY 10021, USA*

With the exception of distant metastases, the single most important prognostic factor in the treatment of patients with squamous cell carcinoma (SCC) of the head and neck is the status of cervical lymph nodes [1]. The presence of even a single lymph node, with metastatic cancer, reduces survival by 50% and contralateral or bilateral nodal involvement reduces survival by an additional 50% [2]. Thus, appropriate management of cervical lymph nodes is extremely crucial in the overall treatment strategy for patients with SCC of the upper aerodigestive tract. The incidence of microscopic metastases in a clinically negative neck can be as high as 25%, making elective treatment of cervical nodes an integral part of the care of high risk patients with head and neck cancer [3].

Classical radical neck dissection (RND) remained the standard practice for management of lymph node metastasis in the neck for nearly three quarters of the past century. However, the philosophy of surgical management of neck metastases has changed considerably over the past few decades. With better understanding of the patterns of nodal spread and nodal level classification, improved anatomic and functional imaging, importance of extracapsular spread (ECS), and better adjuvant therapies, the routine use of RND has been replaced with functional (FND), modified radical (MRND), and selective (SND) neck dissections, to preserve vital structures in the neck and achieve better functional results [4–6]. This article discusses the evolution of neck dissection in the management of cervical lymph nodes in patients with head and neck cancer.

* Corresponding author.
E-mail address: shahj@mskcc.org (J.P. Shah).

History of neck dissection

Maximilian Joseph von Chelius in the mid-nineteenth century stated, "...the neighbouring lymphatics and glands become hard and painful ... once the growth in the mouth has spread to the submaxillary gland, complete removal of the disease is impossible" [7]. Even though Chelius approached neck node metastasis as an incurable situation, Warren recommended "excision of submandibular glands," to control oral cancer [8]. In 1880, Theodore Kocher described the submandibular triangle dissection along with removal of tongue cancer and the upper cervical lymph nodes. The classical double trifurcate incision practiced by him to do the procedure, bears his name, "Kocher incision" [9]. In 1885, Sir Henry Trentham Butlin systematically addressed the upper cervical lymph nodes in tongue cancer [10]; however, he did not remove all of the lymphatic tissue in the neck that was at risk for metastasis. In his Hunterian lecture to the Royal College of Surgeons, in 1898, he proposed excision of upper cervical lymph nodes for tongue cancer.

It was not until 1905, when George Washington Crile Sr., from the Cleveland Clinic, described the first systematic en bloc dissection of lymph nodes in the neck. This, not often quoted, landmark article was entitled "On the surgical treatment of cancer of the head and neck—With a summary of one hundred and twenty-one operations performed upon one hundred and five patients" [11]. It was published in the Transactions of the Southern Surgical and Gynecological Association, with 12 drawings of great clarity and a nine page discussion. Of note, Charles H. Mayo stated, "A large part of abdominal work is recreation as compared with the bulk of what might be called the heavy surgery of the neck, which Dr. Crile has so well described" [12]. The operative technique described became known as the RND. He advocated an en bloc resection of all lymph node bearing tissue, including sacrificing the sternocleidomastoid muscle (SCM), internal jugular vein (IJV), spinal accessory nerve (SAN), submandibular gland, and omohyoid muscle. The RND could be performed in continuity with the primary or as a secondary operation for subsequent metastases. Furthermore, Crile felt that the IJV was the key to cancer dissemination and stated it was essential to sacrifice the vein during the block dissection [12].

In 1906, Crile published his second paper entitled, "Excision of cancer of the head and neck—With a special reference to the plan of dissection based on one hundred and thirty-two operations," in the *Journal of the American Medical Association*. This is the most frequently cited article of Crile with the detailed description of RND [13]. He noted that among the 48 patients who did not have an RND, only nine (19%) were alive in 3 years. However, of the 12 that did have an RND, nine (75%) were alive in 3 years. He concluded that patients who had an RND had a better overall survival than those with lesser operations. The only difference between the two papers relates to the number of cases presented, 121 versus 132, respectively.

Nonetheless, with these two papers, Crile became known as the grandfather of radical neck surgery, and put RND for head and neck cancer on a par with Halsted's radical mastectomy for breast cancer.

Although the name George W. Crile is synonymous with RND, he also proposed preservation of structures like the SAN, SCM, and IJV in patients in whom these structures were not directly involved by the tumor or in patients without palpable nodal disease. The functional outcome and quality of life are directly related to the sacrifice of the SAN. He clearly suspected a biologic difference in tumor behavior and prognosis between patients with and without palpable nodal disease [12]. He is often credited with conceptualizing the modified RND with preservation of the SAN.

The RND remained the gold standard operation for neck metastases for several decades. Blair and Brown, in 1933, advocated routine elective RND with SAN sacrifice to ensure gross total removal of the cervical lymph nodes [14]. Not much is found in the literature after Crile's work until Hayes Martin's classic article was published in *Cancer* in 1951 [15]. As the Chief of the Head and Neck Service at Memorial Hospital for Cancer and Allied Diseases, in New York City, Martin was in the position to perform many RNDs and form very long-lasting opinions about treatment of the neck. He, along with others such as John Conley, were strong proponents of RND for clinically evident neck metastases. Credit goes to him for describing in detail the step-wise procedure of RND. The technique described by Dr. Martin is still followed by many American and international surgeons. Even though RND was quite effective in tumor control, head and neck surgeons appeared to be concerned about the sequelae of RND with sacrifice of SCM, SAN, and IJV, mainly involving shoulder dysfunction, frozen shoulder syndrome, winging of the scapula, cosmetic deformity, chronic pain, and massive facial edema with bilateral RNDs. This led to a gradual change in the philosophy of management of the neck for patients with head and neck cancer.

The first, original, systematic approach to functional neck dissection was published by Osvaldo Suárez, an Argentinean surgeon, in 1963 [16]. Due to the fact that the article was published in Spanish, the operation did not gain popularity in the English-speaking world. Suárez was on the staff of the Department of Otolaryngology at the University of Córdoba Medical School in Argentina. He also worked very closely with Pedro Ara in the Department of Anatomy. Pedro Ara was the famous Spanish anatomist, very popular for having embalmed the corpse of Eva Peron. The FND is not a modification of the RND, but is a different procedure based on the fascial compartments of the neck [17]. Osvaldo Suárez demonstrated that the cervical lymphatics are contained within well defined fascial compartments, separate from muscles, nerves, blood vessels, and other visceral neck structures. He proposed an operation that would allow for removal of all lymphatic tissue in the neck, with preservation of the remaining neck structures, without compromising regional disease control. This would prevent the complications seen with the RND. In 1962, Ettore Bocca had the privilege to observe Suárez in the operating room, and in 1964 he wrote a short paper on the technique [18]. In 1969, during a 2-week course in Europe, both Ettore Bocca from Italy and César Gavilán from Spain, learned the technique directly from Suárez and adopted FND as a new revolutionary approach to the neck [19]. Since then, Bocca and his colleagues have written extensively in the English literature on FND and its outcomes [20–23]. Ettore Bocca receives credit for being the one to introduce FND to the English-speaking world.

A clearer understanding of lymph node drainage patterns led to the development of MRND and SND. During the 1960s, Richard Jesse, Alando Ballantyne, and Robert Byers, surgeons at the M.D. Anderson Cancer Center in Houston, started popularizing the concept of MRND and SND. Only lymph node groups of the neck that were at the highest risk of containing metastases, based on the location of the primary tumor, were removed [24].

The evolution of modern concepts of neck dissection clearly represents an important development in the management of the neck for patients with head and neck cancer. Better understanding of the biology of the disease allows for procedures that address both local control and better functional outcome. Unfortunately, the terminology, "modified" or "functional" neck dissection has led to considerable confusion in the minds of many surgeons. As mentioned above, FND is not a comprehensive operation, it's a conceptual approach to the neck through fascial planes. The extent of the operation has nothing to do with the concept of FND. Therefore, the term MRND is not synonymous with FND. Selective neck dissections represent a modification of FND based on the knowledge of patterns of nodal metastases from different primary sites. In an effort to standardize the nomenclature, the Committee for Head and Neck Surgery and Oncology of the American Academy of Otolaryngology–Head and Neck Surgery published a report in 1991 and a more recent update in 2002 [25]. Neck dissection categories are depicted in Table 1.

Anatomy of lymph node groups and levels

In the current classification schema, the location of cervical lymph node groups is delineated by the level system. This system has been in practice at the Memorial Sloan–Kettering Cancer Center since the 1930s, and has been used worldwide. It is easy to remember and is widely accepted (Fig. 1a). Level I contains lymph nodes in the submental and submandibular triangle. Levels II, III, and IV contain upper, mid, and lower jugular lymph nodes. Level IV nodes include supraclavicular nodes, specifically the scalene group of lymph nodes popularly called Virchow's nodes. Level V includes the posterior triangle group, and level VI includes the central compartment group, which consists of prelaryngeal, pretracheal (Delphian), paratracheal, and tracheoesophageal groove lymph nodes.

Table 1
Classification of neck dissection (AHNS/AAO-HNS)

1991 Classification	2001 Classification
1. Radical neck dissection	1. Radical neck dissection
2. Modified radical neck dissection	2. Modified radical neck dissection
3. Selective neck dissection	3. Selective neck dissection: each variation
a. Supraomohyoid	is depicted by "SND" and the use of
b. Lateral	parentheses to denote the levels or
c. Posterolateral	sublevels removed
d. Anterior	
4. Extended neck dissection	4. Extended neck dissection

Abbreviations: AHNS/AAO-HNS, Committee for Head and Neck Surgery and Oncology of the American Academy of Otolaryngology–Head and Neck Surgery; SND, selective neck dissection.

Data from Ferlito A, Robbins KT, Rinaldo A. Neck Dissection: historical perspective. J Laryngol Otol 2004;118:403–5.

Recently, level I, II, and V nodes have been subclassified into IA, IB, IIA, IIB, VA, and VB (Fig. 1b). Level IA includes submental nodes and Level IB includes submandibular lymph nodes. Level IIA includes lymph nodes below the SAN, and level IIB includes nodes above it. Level VA includes the posterior triangle spinal accessory nodes, and level VB includes the transverse cervical and supraclavicular nodes. The structures defining the anatomic boundaries of the neck levels and sublevels are summarized in Table 2.

Patterns of nodal metastasis

The patterns of nodal metastasis have been extremely well described by Lindberg and Byers and collegues from the M.D. Anderson Cancer Center

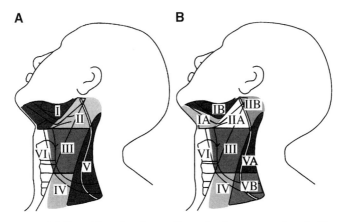

Fig. 1. (*A*) Memorial Sloan–Kettering Cancer Center leveling system of cervical lymph nodes. (*B*) Current modification of leveling system.

Table 2
Anatomical landmarks for the neck levels and sublevels

Level	Superior	Inferior	Anterior (medial)	Posterior (lateral)
IA	Symphysis of mandible	Hyoid bone	Anterior belly of contralateral digastric muscle	Anterior belly of ipsilateral digastric muscle
IB	Mandibular body	Posterior belly of digastric muscle	Anterior belly of digastric muscle	Stylohyoid muscle
IIA	Skull base	Horizontal plane—inferior body of the hyoid bone	Stylohyoid muscle	Vertical plane—spinal accessory nerve
IIB	Skull Base	Horizontal plane—inferior body of the hyoid bone	Vertical plane—spinal accessory nerve	Lateral border of the sternocleidomastoid muscle
III	Horizontal plane—inferior body of the hyoid bone	Horizontal plane—inferior border of the cricoid cartilage	Lateral border of the sternohyoid muscle	Lateral border of the sternocleidomastoid or cervical plexus sensory branches
IV	Horizontal plane—inferior border of the cricoid cartilage	Clavicle	Lateral border of the sternohyoid muscle	Lateral border of the sternocleidomastoid or cervical plexus sensory branches
VA	Convergence of the sternocleidomastoid and trapezius muscles	Horizontal plane—inferior border of the cricoid cartilage	Posterior border of the sternocleidomastoid or cervical plexus sensory branches	Anterior border of the trapezius muscle
VB	Horizontal plane—inferior border of the cricoid cartilage	Clavicle	Posterior border of the sternocleidomastoid or cervical plexus sensory branches	Anterior border of the trapezius muscle
VI	Hyoid bone	Sternum	Common carotid artery	Common carotid artery

[26,27] and Shah from Memorial Sloan–Kettering Cancer Center [28]. Dissemination of metastatic cancer to regional lymph nodes from primary sites in the upper aerodigestive tract occurs in a predictable and sequential fashion [9]. Skip metastases occur very rarely. Sequential progression of disease from level I to V, has prognostic influence, with decreasing survival and worsening outcome in oral cancer. Lymph node metastasis at levels IV and V generally have the worst outcome, with a high incidence of local recurrence and distant metastasis.

The incidence of cervical nodal metastasis depends on characteristics of the primary head and neck tumor. The primary site, size, T stage, location, depth of infiltration, and histology are all important factors influencing the risk of metastatic spread. In general, T stage usually reflects tumor burden or invasiveness, and therefore the risk of nodal metastases increases with increasing T stage of the primary tumor at any site. T1, T2, and T3 tongue cancers have an incidence of cervical nodal disease in the range of 30%, 50%, and 70%, respectively [29]. Tumors of the tongue and floor of mouth greater than 8 mm thick have ~41% risk of occult metastasis. The incidence of cervical nodal disease increases as the location of the primary tumor moves from the anterior to the posterior sites of the oral cavity and oropharynx. Lesions of the tonsil and base of tongue have a very high incidence of metastasis to the neck, and tumors of the hypopharynx universally have metastatic nodal disease. Interestingly, the free border of the true vocal cord has sparse lymphatics; thus, early glottic carcinoma usually never presents with neck node metastasis. However, as the location of the primary tumor in the larynx moves peripherally to the false vocal cords and aryepiglottic folds, the incidence of nodal metastasis increases. In the oral cavity, the tongue has the highest incidence of lymph node metastasis, whereas the hard palate and the lip rarely present with cervical lymph node disease. Certain histomorphologic features of the primary tumor also increase the risk of nodal metastasis. For example, endophytic tumors are more inclined to metastasize when compared with exophytic tumors. In general, if the risk of occult metastases exceeds 15% to 20%, then elective treatment of regional lymph nodes is recommended due to its significantly adverse impact on prognosis [30].

Location of the metastasis is mainly based on the primary site. Lesions of the oral cavity usually metastasize to levels I, II, and III. The recent addition of sublevel IA is useful in that metastasis to this area is very rare. Surgeons may opt to leave level IA out of their dissection unless dealing with primary tumors of the lip or anterior floor of mouth. Primary tumors of the larynx and pharynx commonly metastasize to levels II, III, and IV.

Based on the leveling system and subclassification, one can determine the extent of node dissection based on the above-mentioned characteristics of the primary tumor and patterns of nodal metastasis.

Staging of cervical lymph nodes and prognostic factors

The American Joint Committee on Cancer and the International Union Against Cancer have agreed upon a uniform staging system for cervical lymph nodes. The staging system is shown in Table 3. The N staging system simply reflects the volume of tumor burden in regional lymphatics, which is directly linked to prognosis of the patient. The prognosis worsens with increasing N stage. However, there are other prognostic factors pertaining to lymph nodes that are not included in the current N staging system. These include the location of involved lymph nodes, presence of ECS, perineural, and perivascular infiltration, and presence of tumor emboli in regional lymphatics/subdermal extension of the disease, which are all poor prognostic factors. Patients with ECS have a high incidence of local recurrence and distant metastasis. The incidence of ECS can be as high as 30% in patients with N1 disease, 50% to 70% in patients with N2, and nearly 100% in patients with N3 disease. This is also more common in certain tumors, such as hypopharynx and base of tongue [9].

Classification of neck dissection

The RND is considered the index procedure for cervical lymphadenectomy, with all other operations representing one or more alterations of this procedure. The MRND involves preservation of one or more nonlymphatic structures routinely removed in a RND. Traditionally, MRND is divided into type I (preservation of the SAN), type II (preservation of SAN and SCM), and type III (preservation of SCM, SAN, and IJV). The SND involves excision of select lymph node groups/levels, leaving others routinely removed in RND. Selective lymph node dissections have been divided into supraomohyoid neck dissection (levels I, II, and III), anterolateral or jugular neck dissection (levels II, III, and IV), posterolateral neck dissection

Table 3
N staging of lymph node metastasis from squamous cell carcinoma of the head and neck except nasopharynx (AJCC/UICC, 2002)

Nx	Regional lymph nodes cannot be assessed
N0	No regional lymph node metastasis
N1	Metastasis in a single ipsilateral lymph node, <3 cm in greatest dimension
N2a	Metastasis in a single ipsilateral lymph node, >3 cm but <6 cm in greatest dimension
N2b	Metastases in multiple ipsilateral lymph nodes, none >6 cm in greatest dimension
N2c	Metastases in bilateral or contralateral lymph nodes, none >6 cm in greatest dimension
N3	Metastasis in a lymph node >6 cm in greatest dimension

Abbreviation: AJCC/UICC, American Joint Committee on Cancer and the International Union Against Cancer.

Data from American Joint Committee on Cancer. AJCC cancer staging handbook. 6th edition. New York: Springer; 2002.

(levels II, III, IV, V, and suboccipital nodes), and central compartment dissection (level VI). However, to better standardize the many different variations, SND is defined by the use of parentheses to denote the levels or sublevels removed. Extended neck dissection is defined as the removal of additional lymph node groups or nonlymphatic structures relative to the RND. For example, skin, platysma, cranial nerves, posterior belly of the digastric muscle, external or common carotid artery, styloid musculature, and other lymph node groups are all additional structures that may be sacrificed in an extended neck dissection.

Radical neck dissection

The RND (Fig. 2) refers to the comprehensive removal of all ipsilateral cervical lymph node groups. The boundaries include superiorly, the inferior border of the mandible; inferiorly, the clavicle; medially, the sternohyoid muscle, hyoid bone, and contralateral anterior belly of the digastric muscle; and laterally, the anterior border of the trapezius muscle. Included in the dissection are levels I through V, SCM, IJV, SAN, and submandibular salivary gland. Although the RND is not commonly used today, it may still have the following important indications [9]:

1. Upper neck N3 disease
2. Bulky metastatic disease near the SAN
3. Tumor directly involving the SAN
4. Recurrent disease in the neck after previous dissection
5. Recurrent disease in the neck after previous radiation therapy
6. Involvement of platysma or skin
7. Clinical signs of gross extranodal disease

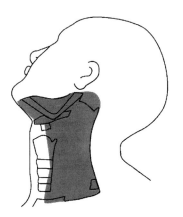

Lymph nodes dissected
• Level I
• Level II
• Level III
• Level IV
• Level V

Other structures excised
• Sternocleidomastoid muscle
• Internal jugular vein
• Spinal accessory nerve
• Submandibular gland

Fig. 2. Classic radical neck dissection.

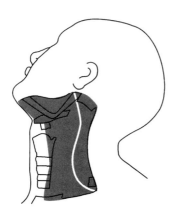

Lymph nodes dissected
• Level I
• Level II
• Level III
• Level IV
• Level V

Other structures excised
• Sternocleidomastoid muscle
• Internal jugular vein
• Submandibular gland

Structures preserved
• Spinal accessory nerve

Fig. 3. Modified radical neck dissection with preservation of SAN (type I).

Modified radical neck dissection

The MRND (Figs. 3, 4, and 5) refers to the removal of lymph node levels I through V, with the preservation of one or more of the nonlymphatic structures that are routinely removed in a RND. In describing the operation, the structure preserved should be specifically named (ex. MRND with preservation of SAN). The indications for a MRND are similar to RND. It is difficult to justify the routine sacrifice of an uninvolved SAN, when uninvolved hypoglossal and vagus nerves are spared. Currently, the most

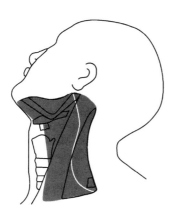

Lymph nodes dissected
• Level I
• Level II
• Level III
• Level IV
• Level V

Other structures excised
• Internal jugular vein
• Submandibular gland

Structures preserved
• Sternocleidomastoid muscle
• Spinal accessory nerve

Fig. 4. Modified radical neck dissection with preservation of SCM and SAN (type II).

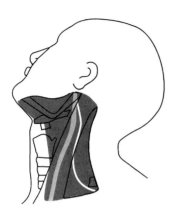

Lymph nodes dissected
- Level I
- Level II
- Level III
- Level IV
- Level V

Other structures excised
- Submandibular gland

Structures preserved
- Internal jugular vein
- Sternocleidomastoid muscle
- Spinal accessory nerve

Fig. 5. Modified radical neck dissection with preservation of IJV, SCM, and SAN (type III).

frequently employed MRND for SSC with palpable neck metastases is MRND preserving the SAN (type I).

Modified neck dissection preserving the SCM, SAN and IJV (type III) is generally recommended for metastatic differentiated carcinoma of the thyroid gland. The indolent and nonaggressive biologic behavior of well-differentiated thyroid cancer justifies the preservation of these structures.

Selective neck dissection

The SND refers to the selective removal of one or more of the nodal groups/levels. It is commonly used for accurate staging and treatment of the clinically disease free (N0) neck at risk of harboring occult micrometastasis. The lymph node levels removed are based on the location primary tumor and the patterns of nodal metastasis as mentioned above. The selective removal of lymph node groups that are at the greatest risk for harboring metastatic disease represents one of the most significant paradigm shifts in the management of head and neck cancer. This treatment philosophy has been applied mostly to patients with a N0 neck; however, SND is also being performed in select patients for the treatment of N + neck [31,32]. The named SNDs have been replaced by descriptive nomenclature that state the levels removed.

Selective neck dissection for oral cavity cancer: supraomohyoid (levels I–III) and extended supraomohyoid neck dissection (levels I–IV)

The nodal groups at risk in oral cavity cancer include levels I, II, and III. The procedure of choice would be SND I–III (Fig. 6). There is also some data that suggests increased risk of level IV involvement in anterolateral tongue lesions [33]. In such instances, the procedure of choice would be

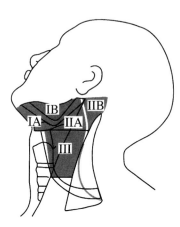

Lymph nodes dissected
• Level I
• Level II
• Level III

Other structures excised
• Submandibular gland

Fig. 6. Selective lymph node dissection levels I–III (supraomohyoid).

SND I–IV (Fig. 7). For lesions in the midline, involving the floor of mouth or ventral tongue, lymph nodes on both sides are at risk for nodal metastasis and bilateral SND I–III may be indicated. The neck dissection may be performed in conjunction with excision of the primary tumor, either in continuity in a monobloc fashion or as a discontinuous procedure where the primary tumor is removed through a per oral approach.

Selective neck dissection for oropharyngeal, laryngeal, and hypopharyngeal cancer: jugular (anterolateral) neck dissection (levels II–IV)

Based on the knowledge of patterns of nodal metastasis, tumors affecting these sites may metastasize to lymph nodes in levels II–IV. The procedure of

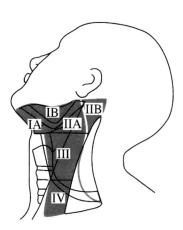

Lymph nodes dissected
• Level I
• Level II
• Level III
• Level IV

Other structures excised
• Submandibular gland

Fig. 7. Selective lymph node dissection levels I–IV (extended supraomohyoid).

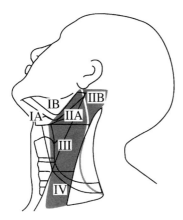

Lymph nodes dissected

• Level II
• Level III
• Level IV

Fig. 8. Selective lymph node dissection levels II–IV (jugular/anterolateral).

choice in these cases would be SND II–IV (Fig. 8). Tumors in these sites often cross the midline and the procedure of choice becomes bilateral SND II–IV in cases where the neck is managed surgically. Level IIB is at greater risk for metastatic disease with oropharyngeal lesions. Thus, with tumors involving the larynx or hypopharynx where Level IIB is excluded, the procedure would be designated SND levels IIA, III, and IV. In cases where hypopharyngeal and laryngeal tumors extend below the level of the glottis, lymph nodes from level VI are usually included in the neck dissection [34]. The procedure would be designated SND II–IV, and VI.

Selective neck dissection for midline anterior lower neck cancer: central compartment neck dissection (level VI)

This procedure is usually indicated for tumors arising in the thyroid gland, cervical trachea, cervical esophagus, and laryngeal and hypopharyngeal tumors extending below the level of the glottic larynx. It involves removal of all the lymph nodes in level VI (Fig. 9). In cases where lymph nodes extend into the mediastinum, the dissection would include SND VI, superior mediastinal lymph nodes. For thyroid tumors with lateral neck metastases, the procedure of choice would be SND II–V, and VI.

Selective neck dissection: posterolateral type (levels II–V, postauricular, suboccipital)

This type of neck dissection is primarily used for nodal metastases associated with cutaneous malignancies of the posterior scalp and neck. The neck dissection is designed to encompass all of the lymph nodes of the posterior and lateral compartments of the neck, including suboccipital lymph nodes (Fig. 10).

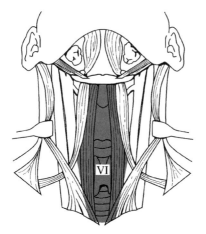

Lymph nodes dissected

Level VI

• Delphian

• Perithyroid

• Tracheo-esophageal groove

Fig. 9. Selective lymph node dissection level VI (central compartment).

Extended neck dissection

Extended neck dissection refers to a procedure more extensive than a RND, where additional lymph node groups or nonlymphatic structures are removed. Examples of such lymph node groups include retropharyngeal, parapharyngeal, superior mediastinal, perifacial, and axillary nodes. Non-lymphatic structures can include skin, platysma, hypoglossal or vagus nerve, posterior belly of the digastric muscle, external or common carotid artery, or styloid musculature (Fig. 11).

Selective neck dissection: future directions

A possible alternative to elective surgical treatment of cervical lymph nodes for oral carcinoma is lymphoscintigraphy and sentinel node biopsy.

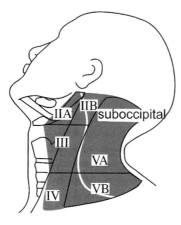

Lymph nodes dissected

• Level II

• Level III

• Level IV

• Level V

• Suboccipital triangle

Fig. 10. Selective lymph node dissection levels II–V, postauricular, suboccipital (posterolateral).

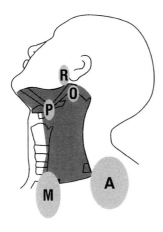

Additional lymph nodes dissected

• R- retropharyngeal
• P- parapharyngeal
• M- mediastinal
• A- axillary

or

**Other non-lymphatic
structures removed**

• O- Cranial nerves, carotid artery,
    muscles, skin, etc.

Fig. 11. Extended radical neck dissection.

This technique, which was championed by Morton [35] for extremity and truncal melanoma, has already become an accepted staging tool for breast carcinoma and cutaneous melanoma. Sentinel lymph node biopsy is based on the same principles as SND, in that lymphatic metastases do not occur randomly, but rather predictably, in a stepwise manner. The use of sentinel lymph node biopsy in head and neck mucosal SCC may ultimately allow adequate staging of the N0 neck and help direct elective treatment strategies. It has the potential of avoiding either undertreatment or overtreatment of the neck [36]. It should be noted that sentinel lymph node biopsy for head and neck mucosal SCC is currently only an investigational tool.

Summary

The philosophy of management of metastatic disease in the neck has changed considerably over the past few decades. With better understanding of the patterns of lymph node metastases, leading to subclassification of levels and understanding the importance of prognostic factors such as ECS and perineural invasion, we have been able to preserve uninvolved lymphatic and nonlymphatic structures. The RND, which has been the standard of care for management of neck metastasis, has essentially been replaced by MRND and SND. The improved quality of life and functional outcomes have helped guide this evolution. More extensive surgery does not necessarily equate to a better oncologic outcome, and less can often mean more [1]. Special techniques such as ultrasound, ultrasound-guided needle biopsy, and sentinel node biopsy have the potential to further refine our surgical expertise to eradicate the cancer, preserve function and cosmesis, and maintain excellent oncologic outcomes.

References

[1] Ferlito A, Rinaldo A, Robbins KT, et al. Changing concepts in the surgical management of the cervical node metastasis. Oral Oncol 2003;39(5):429–35.

[2] Myers EN, Fagan JJ. Treatment of the N + neck in squamous cell carcinoma of the upper aerodigestive tract. Otolaryngol Clin North Am 1998;31:671–86.

[3] Houck JR, Medina JE. Management of cervical lymph nodes in squamous carcinomas of the head and neck. Semin Surg Oncol 1995;11:228–39.

[4] American Joint Committee on Cancer. AJCC cancer staging handbook. 6th edition. New York: Springer; 2002.

[5] Medina JE. A rational classification of neck dissections. Otolaryngol Head Neck Surg 1989; 100:169–76.

[6] Byers RM. Modified neck dissection. A study of 967 cases from 1970 to 1980. Am J Surg 1985;150:414–21.

[7] Chelius JM, South JF. A system of surgery. Tr. from the German and accompanied with additional notes and observations by John F. South. Philadelphia: Lea & Blanchard; 1847. Vol. III, p. 515.

[8] Warren JC. Surgical observations on tumours, with cases and operations. London: John Churchill; 1839.

[9] Shaha AR. Radical neck dissection. Oper Tech Gen Surg 2004;6(2):72–82.

[10] Butlin HT. Diseases of the tongue. London: Cassell & Co.; 1885.

[11] Crile GW. On the surgical treatment of cancer of the head and neck—with a summary of one hundred and twenty-one operations performed upon one hundred and five patients. Trans South Surg Gynecol Assoc 1905;18:108–27.

[12] Ferlito A, Robbins KT, Rinaldo A. Neck dissection: historical perspective. J Laryngol Otol 2004;118(6):403–5.

[13] Crile GW. Excision of cancer of the head and neck—with a special reference to the plan of dissection based on one hundred and thirty-two operations. JAMA 1906;47:1780–6.

[14] Blair VP, Brown JP. The treatment of cancerous or potentially cancerous cervical lymph nodes. Ann Surg 1933;98:650–61.

[15] Martin HE, Del Valle B, Ehrlich H, et al. Neck dissection. Cancer 1951;4:441–99.

[16] Suárez O. El problema de las metastasis linfáticas y alejadas del cáncer de laringe e hipofaringe. Rev Otorrinolaringol 1963;23:83–99.

[17] Ferlito A, Gavilan J, Buckley JG, et al. Functional neck dissection: Fact and fiction. Head Neck 2001;23(9):804–8.

[18] Bocca E. Évidement "fonctionel" du cou dans la thérapie de principe des metastases ganglionnaires du cancer du larynx (introduction à la présentation d'un film). J Fr Otorhinolaryngol 1964;13:721–3.

[19] Ferlito A, Rinaldo A. Osvaldo Suarez: often-forgotten father of functional neck dissection (in the non-Spanish-speaking literature). Laryngoscope 2004;114(7):1177–8.

[20] Bocca E, Pignataro O, Oldini C, et al. Functional neck dissection: an evaluation and review of 843 cases. Laryngoscope 1984;94(7):942–5.

[21] Bocca E, Pignataro O, Sasaki CT. Functional neck dissection. A description of operative technique. Arch Otolaryngol 1980;106(9):524–7.

[22] Bocca E, Pignataro O. A conservation technique in radical neck dissection. Ann Otol Rhinol Laryngol 1967;76(5):975–87.

[23] Bocca E. Supraglottic laryngectomy and functional neck dissection. J Laryngol Otol 1966; 80(8):831–8.

[24] Jesse RH, Ballantyne AJ, Larson D. Radical or modified neck dissection: a therapeutic dilemma. Am J Surg 1978;136:516–9.

[25] Robbins KT, Clayman G, Levine PA, et al. Neck dissection classification update: revisions proposed by the American Head and Neck Society and the American Academy of

Otolaryngology-Head and Neck Surgery. Arch Otolaryngol Head Neck Surg 2002;128(7): 751–8.

[26] Lindberg R. Distribution of cervical lymph node metastases from squamous cell carcinoma of the upper respiratory and digestive tracts. Cancer 1972;29(6):1446–9.

[27] Byers RM, Wolf PF, Ballantyne AJ. Rationale for elective modified neck dissection. Head Neck Surg 1988;10(3):160–7.

[28] Shah JP. Patterns of cervical lymph node metastasis from squamous carcinomas of the upper aerodigestive tract. Am J Surg 1990;160(4):405–9.

[29] Spiro RH, Huvos AG, Wong GY, et al. Predictive value of tumor thickness in squamous carcinoma confined to the tongue and floor of mouth. Am J Surg 1986;152:345–50.

[30] Shah JP, Patel SG. Cervical lymph nodes. In: Head and neck surgery and oncology. 3rd edition. St. Louis: Mosby; 2003. p. 353–94.

[31] Traynor SJ, Cohen JI, Gray J, et al. Selective neck dissection and the management of the node-positive neck. Am J Surg 1996;172(6):654–7.

[32] Pellitteri PK, Robbins KT, Neuman T. Expanded application of selective neck dissection with regard to nodal status. Head Neck 1997;19(4):260–5.

[33] Byers RM, Weber RS, Andrews T, et al. Frequency and therapeutic implications of "skip metastases" in the neck from squamous carcinoma of the oral tongue. Head Neck 1997;19: 14–9.

[34] Brentani RR, Kowalski LP, Soares JF, et al. End results of a prospective trial on elective lateral neck dissection vs type III modified radical neck dissection in the management of supraglottic and transglottic carcinomas. Head Neck 1999;21:694–702.

[35] Morton DL, Wen DR, Wong JH, et al. Technical details of the intraoperative lymphatic mapping for early stage melanoma. Arch Surg 1992;127:392–9.

[36] Rigual NR, Wiseman SM. Neck dissection: current concepts and future directions. Surg Oncol Clin N Am 2004;13:151–66.

ELSEVIER
SAUNDERS

Surg Oncol Clin N Am
14 (2005) 479–498

SURGICAL
ONCOLOGY CLINICS
OF NORTH AMERICA

The Evolution of Surgery for Breast Cancer

David P. Winchester, MD, FACS[a,b],
Lucrecia Trabanino, MD[c,d],
Marvin J. Lopez, MD[c,d],*

[a]Department of Surgery, Evanston Northwestern Healthcare,
2650 Ridge Avenue, Evanston, IL 60201, USA
[b]Department of Surgery, Northwestern University Medical School,
251 East Huron Street, Galter 3-150, Chicago, IL 60611-2950, USA
[c]Tufts University School of Medicine, 136 Harrison Avenue, Boston, MA 02111, USA
[d]Department of Surgery, Caritas St. Elizabeth's Medical Center of Boston,
736 Cambridge Street, Boston, MA 02135, USA

Although cancer of the breast was documented 5000 years ago as is seen in the Edwin Smith papyrus, surgical treatment for this disease could only be described as primitive. In the preanesthesia era surgical treatment consisted of tumor cauterization for exposed, ulcerated, locally advanced disease, or, for long-neglected tumors, guillotine-type knife amputation of the breast [1]. One can imagine the massive bleeding, the pain, and the suffering caused by the brutal treatment. For most of the women, severe anemia and infected open flesh resulted in septicemia and death. For those who survived the treatment, metastatic disease led to death in a few months. The serious student of breast disease will be interested in John Brown's [2] (1810–1882) vivid and horrific 1858 account of a breast surgical intervention performed by James Syme (1799–1870), father in-law of Lord Lister, and famous for the amputation technique that bears his name.

In the mid-nineteenth century, the European schools of surgery, especially those in Germany and Great Britain, provided the impetus for the study of breast disease and the birth of modern surgery. Surgical scholars replaced barber-surgeons. Antisepsis and the introduction of anesthesia in the mid-1800s revolutionized surgery, while histopathology

* Corresponding author. Department of Surgery, Caritas St. Elizabeth's Medical Center of Boston, 736 Cambridge Street, Boston, MA 02135.
 E-mail address: Marvin.Lopez.MD@caritaschristi.org (M.J. Lopez).

1055-3207/05/$ - see front matter © 2005 Elsevier Inc. All rights reserved.
doi:10.1016/j.soc.2005.04.006
surgonc.theclinics.com

and long-term observations in large numbers of patients provided the modern basis for breast surgery.

These observations by the most prominent physicians of the time dealt principally with detailed clinical and histopathologic observations and very little with effective forms of treatment. Theodor Billroth, one the most eminent European surgeons of the late 1800s, dedicates 12 pages to breast cancer in his 664-page book *General Surgical Pathology and Therapeutics*, published in 1871. Only a few comments are made regarding surgery of breast cancer. The reader of this classic treatise will appreciate the sad state of treatment for breast cancer at the time. Billroth writes: "Before passing to the choice of these [therapeutic] methods, we must consider the question, whether it is advisable to operate at all, even if it can be done easily and without danger to life, for the views of experienced surgeons differ on this point. Some surgeons never operate for cancer. They assert that the operation is always in vain, because the disease recurs; if the recurring tumors be operated on, new recurrence takes place the sooner." It is not difficult to understand Billroth's position on the extent of surgery when he writes: "In reply to the question, whether carcinoma should ever be operated on, we may say that operation probably has no direct influence on the diathesis, and that the operation, if done at all, must be done for other reasons." Billroth identified palliation and local disease control as the "indirect" benefit of surgical extirpation of cancerous breasts [3]. Table 1 depicts several European seminal contributions in the study of breast cancer during the later part of the nineteenth century.

Table 1
Evolution of radical surgery for breast cancer: important contributions in the nineteenth century

1800–1850	Observations on the pathology and natural history of breast cancer/primitive amputations of the breast in the preanesthetic, preanesthesia era
1822	Elliott reported first microscopic examinations of a metastatic lymph node
1856	Paget published observations from 374 cases. Questioned the value of surgery for cure of breast cancer. Described the infiltrating carcinoma of the breast and nipple that bears his name.
1867	Moore published a paper on "the influence of inadequate operations on the cure of cancer." The era of radical surgery begins.
1867	Lister writes on antiseptic principles, supports Moore's radical surgical approach in the treatment of breast cancer.
1875	Volkmann removes entire breast and pectoral fascia.
1877	Banks advocates routine removal of axillary lymph nodes
1878	Billroth performs lumpectomy for early breast cancer, but advocates resection of the entire breast and axillary lymph nodes for most cases.
1894	Halsted publishes results of the "complete operation" in 50 cases. Removes breast en bloc with pectoralis major muscle and axillary lymph nodes.
1894	Meyer described a similar technique advocating the removal of the pectoralis minor muscle as well.
1891	Welch first to employ frozen section in the diagnosis of breast cancer.

Development and stardardization of radical mastectomy

In the United States surgery came of age after the introduction of anesthesia by Morton at the Massachusetts General Hospital in 1846. Several American surgeons, principally from the northeastern cities of Philadelphia, Baltimore, New York, and Boston, left their indelible mark in breast surgery during the latter half of the nineteenth century. Pancoast, as early as 1844, performed an operation that was indistinguishable from later descriptions of an en bloc resection of the breast and axillary contents [4]. Opinions regarding the aggressiveness with which breast cancer should be treated varied in American surgery. Samuel D. Gross favored a conservative approach, a simple mastectomy with primary skin closure, whereas his son, Samuel W. Gross, preferred a more radical treatment that included excising the pectoral fascia, the axillary lymph nodes, all of the breast skin, and leaving the open wound to granulate.

William S. Halsted was influenced by the German school of surgery to develop an approach to breast cancer that was more aggressive than those used by Billroth and Volkmann. Halsted attributed the high local recurrence rate of the German surgeons to failure to obtain adequate surgical resection margins. Thus, he advocated the routine use of en bloc resection of the pectoralis major muscle, for he repeatedly encountered tumor deposits near or through the fascia. His fame derived not from the development of a radical operation or improvement in long-term survival, but from the impact of what he called the "complete method" (referring to radical mastectomy) on local control of the disease. He wrote: "The efficiency of an operation is measured truer in terms of local recurrence than of ultimate cure. For some lives are rescued only by repeated operations for local recurrence, and others, free from local recurrence, are lost from internal metastases" [5]. The dismal survival of breast cancer patients is evidenced by his 1894 report of 3-year survival results among the best surgeons of the day ranging from 4% for Billroth to 30% for Bergman. Halsted later reported his own overall 5-year survival rate of 45% and 72% for patients with node-negative breast cancer [6].

Fig. 1 depicts the local recurrence rates during the late 1800s. Data from well-known German surgeons are compared with Dr. Halsted's first report of 50 cases. The dramatic reduction in local recurrence rates was attributed to the improved surgical resection margins of the radical mastectomy. Fig. 2 allows a comparison of Halsted's first 50 cases, which he described with sufficient detail to determine the T and the N class, with the stage distribution 100 years later at the Center for Breast Care of Caritas Saint Elizabeth's Medical Center, a tertiary care university-affiliated community hospital in Boston (Fig. 3). It is remarkable that in Halsted's report, there were no in situ or even stage I breast cancer cases and only 8% of stage II breast cancers. Not surprisingly, in the era before radiation therapy and systemic treatment of breast cancer, his operation was a major contribution

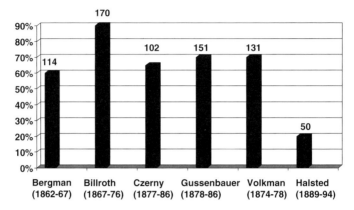

Fig. 1. Nineteenth century breast cancer surgery: local recurrence rates. (*From* Halsted WS. The results of operations for the cure of cancer of the breast performed at the Johns Hopkins Hospital from June 1889 to January 1894. Johns Hopkins Hospital Rep 1894–1895;4:297–31, with permission.)

to the care of patients who invariably presented with locally advanced disease. Although more recent publications on breast preserving treatment have cast Dr. Halsted's contribution in a negative light, when the operation was developed, it was the only choice for local control. For example, a photograph (Fig. 4) of one of Halsted's patients shows an obvious T4, stage IIIb carcinoma of the breast that had to be resected with a vast area of skin. It is also tempting to speculate that the tumor proximity to the pectoral muscle demanded better margins than the pectoral fascia alone could provide; thus, his adherence to the precept of routine sacrifice of a large

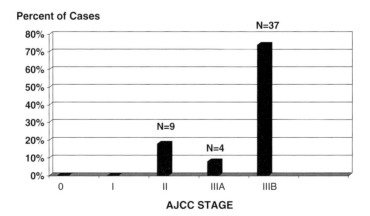

Fig. 2. Clinical stage of breast cancer in 50 patients operated upon by Halsted from 1889–1894. (*From* Halsted WS. The results of operations for the cure of cancer of the breast performed at the Johns Hopkins Hospital from June 1889 to January 1894. Johns Hopkins Hospital Rep 1894–1895;4:297–31, with permission.)

Percent of Cases

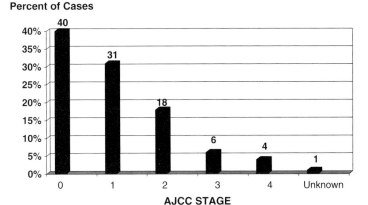

Fig. 3. Caritas St. Elizabeth's Medical Center of Boston. Distribution by American Joint Committee on Cancer stage analytic breast cancer cases, 1998.

portion of the breast skin, the pectoralis major muscle, and the axillary lymph nodes.

A vast body of information on breast cancer surgery permeated the American and European literature in the first 2 decades of the twentieth century. Although it is not difficult to find early attempts at breast preservation, the great majority of operations for breast cancer employed the radical mastectomy as modified by Meyer. His operation, published only days after Halsted's, included resection of the pectoralis minor muscle. The Halsted-Meyer operation became better known in the mid to late twentieth century as the classic Halsted Radical Mastectomy. However important

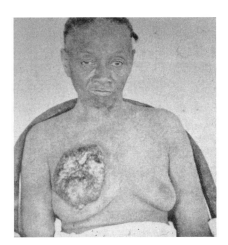

Fig. 4. Halsted's patient with locally advanced stage breast cancer circa 1885. (*Reproduced from* Halsted WS. Surgical Papers. In: The Classics of Surgery Library, vol. 2. Birmingham (AL): 1984; with permission.)

Halsted's contribution was, his use of radical surgery was by no means singular. In a symposium on breast cancer at the May 8, 1907 meeting of the American Surgical Association, papers were read by several luminaries, among them Albert J. Ochsner of Chicago (98 cases), Nathan Jacobson of Syracuse, NY (164 cases), John Chadwick Oliver of Cincinnati (35 cases), and Arthur Tracy Cabot of Boston (42 cases). According to these papers, locally advanced breast cancer was prevalent, radical mastectomy was most often performed to alleviate suffering, the operative mortality by the turn of the century had dropped from 4% to 10% to less than 1%, and the survival rates were now measured in 5-year terms instead of 3 years as proposed by Volkmann in the late 1800s.

During the first half of the twentieth century, little changed in the epidemiology of breast cancer and primary therapy with radical mastectomy. Some controversy not withstanding, the standard of care for operable breast cancer did not appreciably change until after World War II, when surgery was extended beyond the confines of radical mastectomy. Halsted reported dissecting the supraclavicular lymph node region, probably prompted by the presence of adenopathy, in a futile effort to prevent further cancer spread. However, in a 1950 report by Taylor and Wallace describing a 50-year experience with breast cancer treatment at the Massachusetts General Hospital, Owen Wangensteen, one of the great American surgical leaders of the twentieth century, commented that "Today, it should be said, I believe, the Halsted operation for cancer of the breast is outmoded; it is not radical enough; it is an incomplete operation for cancer of the breast in patients exhibiting axillary metastases. The extension of the conventional Halsted operation as I have been doing it consists of the following additional items done simultaneously: (1) a supraclavicular dissection, performed with the clavicle retracted laterally; (2) excision of the internal mammary chain of vessels and the intercostal lymph nodes lying in juxtaposition to the vessels; it has been feasible to remove, too, the contralateral chain of internal mammary vessels; and (3) a mediastinal dissection" [7].

Another proponent of more extensive surgery was Jerome A. Urban. Stimulated by the works of Handley in 1927 [8], Neuhof in 1938 [9], and Gardner in 1951 [10], he popularized the supraradical mastectomy in which the internal mammary lymph nodes were also removed. In a 1952 report of 40 patients so treated, the incidence of internal mammary lymph node metastases in patients with breast cancer located medial to the nipple was 47%, but was only 5% in patients with negative axillary lymph nodes even in medial quadrant lesions [11]. Few surgeons embraced this supraradical concept, and it was soon abandoned.

A major contribution to our current understanding of the natural history of breast cancer was made in 1943 by Cushman Haagensen, a life-long student of breast disease, whose criteria of inoperability is a classic in surgical oncology [12]. He recognized that locally advanced breast cancer should not be operated upon because surgical resection did not contribute to survival. The inoperability criteria included breast cancer that ulcerated, became fixed to the chest wall, developed satellite nodules or cutaneous changes associated with the inflammatory-type of breast cancer, and locally advanced axillary lymphadenopathy, such as enlarged lymph nodes that adhered to each other or were fixed to the axillary chest wall. In current staging terminology, these would be patients with stage IIIb breast cancer, similar to those frequently operated by Dr. Halsted.

Early in the twentieth century, the routine use of radiation therapy began as a desperate attempt to control advanced primary or recurrent disease. Its use as prophylaxis dates to the 1920s with the use of radium tubes, the forerunner of brachytherapy. Handley recognized that many of the local failures were supraclavicular and internal mammary, because "recurrence in the axilla after an efficient operation is very rare." With that in mind, he placed four radium tubes near the internal mammary nodal chain and in the supraclavicular region [8]. Nearly 100 years later, prophylactic external beam irradiation, so-called adjuvant, is still used to eliminate recurrence at these nodal sites. Another classic of the radiation oncology literature that had a major impact in treatment decisions for decades was a paper by Baclesse, who advocated local excision of breast cancer followed by "adequate" radiotherapy or treatment by irradiation alone. He claimed results equal to those of radical operations [13,14].

Modified radical mastectomy

We believe that the transition to modified radical mastectomy resulted in part from the advent of external beam radiotherapy as an adjuvant to total mastectomy. Because the success of mastectomy was, and is, measured by the local disease control rates, it follows that chest wall irradiation probably eliminated microscopic disease near or at the pectoral fascia level. A second factor in the transition to modified radical mastectomy was the pro-portionate increase in the incidence of stage I and II breast cancer and relative reduction of locally advanced disease, which resulted in less need to remove the pectoral muscles to obtain adequate surgical resection margins. Murphy and Grace were early opponents of radical mastectomy [15,16].

Patey and associates from England described in 1948 an operation in which the entire breast was removed with the pectoralis minor muscle and the axillary contents, preserving the pectoralis major. Resection of the pectoralis minor facilitates excision of level III axillary lymph nodes. They later reported experience with 146 cases of breast carcinoma so treated between 1930 and 1943. Their results were comparable to those obtained with radical mastectomy [17,18]. The Patey operation remained in vogue primarily in Europe for many years. American surgeons Auchincloss and Madden used a technique that preserved both of the pectoralis muscles [19,20]. In so doing, level III axillary lymph nodes were not dissected. These results from modified breast surgery were corroborated by reports from other institutions [21,22]. All of these retrospective reviews suggested that avoiding level III axillary lymphadenectomy did not affect survival. The Auchincloss-Madden modified radical mastectomy, which dissects level I and II axillary lymph nodes, became the standard of care in North America during the 1970s. It remains the best treatment for primary, early-stage, multicentric breast carcinoma associated with axillary lymph node metastases. The transition in the standard of care from radical to modified radical mastectomy was swift, taking only a few years, as shown by a pattern of care study of the Commission on Cancer of the American College of Surgeons published in 1984 [23]. The classic radical mastectomy for treatment of operable, early stage breast carcinoma was abandoned over a quarter century ago.

Beginning in the 1970s, prospective, randomized clinical trials compared various forms of surgical treatment with and without adjuvant therapy. Two trials of historic importance settled any remaining issues regarding the preferred type of mastectomy. In Manchester, England, a trial that was conducted from 1969 to 1976, randomized 534 patients with stage I and II breast carcinoma to either radical mastectomy (N = 278) or modified radical mastectomy (N = 256). The two groups were comparable in terms of tumor stage distribution. Although the precise lymph node dissection technique in each group is unclear, as is the number of metastatic lymph nodes per patient in relation to each type of mastectomy, it is evident that both procedures cleared at least levels I and II axillary lymph nodes. These investigators found no statistical differences in disease-free survival, local recurrence rates, or overall survival rates [24]. Second, a trial to compare radical to modified radical mastectomy was conducted by Maddox and associates at the University of Alabama from 1975 to 1978. Patients with metastatic axillary lymph nodes were further randomized to receive one of two combinations of chemotherapeutic agents. Although the results showed no statistically significant difference in disease-free survival between the two operative groups, lower local recurrence rates were associated with radical mastectomy at the 5-year follow-up point, and became significant at the 10-year mark [25]. Possibly these more favorable results were because of better surgical resection margins obtained with radical mastectomy.

Yet another classic study was the National Surgical Adjuvant Breast and Bowel Project (NSABP) B-O4. It was a prospective, randomized clinical trial comparing three surgical arms, radical mastectomy, total (simple) mastectomy followed by loco-regional radiation therapy and total mastectomy alone with an axillary dissection performed only when lymph nodes became clinically metastatic. Through 10 years of follow-up, Fisher and associates reported no differences in disease-free survival among the three groups for both node-negative and node-positive breast carcinoma [26].

The era of modified radical mastectomy as the preferred form of treatment for breast cancer was soon challenged by prospective, randomized clinical trials comparing total mastectomy against lumpectomy combined with whole breast irradiation. The advent of sentinel lymph node mapping in the 1990s further reduced the percentage of patients with breast cancer necessitating a modified radical mastectomy.

In 2004, analysis of unpublished tumor registry data from Caritas Saint Elizabeth's Medical Center of Boston for invasive and noninvasive breast cancer revealed that of the patients who had multicentric breast cancer and clinically positive lymph nodes, 5% received the Auchincloss-Madden modified radical mastectomy, 13% were treated with total mastectomy and 82% received lumpectomy plus breast irradiation. Except for the 5% of patients having an en bloc axillary lymphadenectomy as part of the modified radical procedure, sentinel lymph node biopsy was performed in all cases of infiltrating breast carcinoma. Thirteen percent of these patients had lymph node metastasis, half of whom had disease confined to the sentinel lymph node. Today, statistics like these are commonplace in the United States, representing a remarkable change in epidemiology and treatment paradigm for breast cancer since the 1970s. Credit must be given to the many organizations which promoted early breast cancer detection practices in the United States and the thousands of patients who were willing to participate

Table 2
Evolution of surgery for breast cancer: landmark contributions in the twentieth century

1907	Halsted reported results of radical mastectomy and supraclavicular dissection in 119 patients
1912	J.B. Murphy abandons radical mastectomy. His approach marks early attempts at modified radical mastectomy
1913	Solomon describes mammography
1927	Handley reports removal of internal mammary lymph nodes
1938	Gershon-Cohen recommends screening for breast cancer
1943	Haagensen publishes criteria of inoperability for locally advanced breast cancer
1948	Patey describes modified radical mastectomy with removal of the pectoralis minor muscle
1950–1951	Wangensteen and Urban describe an ultraradical approach to breast cancer surgery, removing the internal mammary nodes
1960	Egan defines modern mammography
1963–1965	Auchincloss and Madden describe modified radical mastectomy preserving both pectoral muscles
1971	Fisher and NSABP members launch protocol B-04, comparing radical mastectomy, total mastectomy, plus radiotherapy, and total mastectomy alone for breast carcinoma
1976	NSABP protocol B-06 is initiated. It compares total mastectomy, lumpectomy, plus radiation and lumpectomy alone
1981–1983	Turner and Maddox report on the Manchester and University of Alabama trials of radical versus modified radical mastectomy, showing no difference in survival
1985–1995	Protocols B-04 (10-year results) and B-06 (12-year results) are reported showing no difference in survival
1992–1994	Krag and Guiliano publish individual contributions in the development of sentinel lymph node mapping for breast, based on Morton's pioneering efforts in melanoma

in prospective, randomized clinical trials. Table 2 lists selected important contributions in breast cancer surgery in the twentieth century.

The era of breast preservation in breast cancer surgery

The earliest account of local excision of breast cancer dates back to the Dark Ages. The Greek physician Galen established a medical dogma in the second century A.D., which was to endure for nearly 1000 years. Galen believed that cancer developed because of melancholia, an excess of black bile. Cancer was treated by diet and purgation. Galen made a therapeutic exception for breast cancers he judged to be surgically removable. By his own remarkable description, Galen stated "In all operations we attempt to excise a pathologic tumor in a circle, in the region where it borders on the healthy tissue" [27]. Nearly 2 centuries later, surgeons strive to achieve clear margins with lumpectomy.

In modern days, one of the major barriers to moving from mastectomy to breast-conserving surgery in properly selected patients was the well-documented observation by Gallager [28] that breast cancer was frequently a multicentric disease. This 1969 report from the M.D. Anderson Cancer Center was based upon a meticulous whole-organ sectioning of 60 radical mastectomy specimens. Of the 47 breasts containing invasive carcinomas, 22 involved multiple invasive sites often separated by wide distances. Gallager suggested that these multiple foci resulted from preexisting intraductal carcinoma or spread along periductal lymphatics to form secondary nodules. Gallager concluded that "human mammary carcinoma is not a focal process but a disease which affects breast epithelia diffusely." Findings similar to Gallager's were reported by Qualheim [29] in 1957.

In 1980, Schwartz and associates [30] reported that the incidence of multicentricity in 43 mastectomy specimens examined was 44.2%. They concluded that "These findings suggested that any therapeutic procedure for either invasive or noninvasive ductal carcinoma that does not include total mastectomy may leave behind foci of cancer, which are a threat to the patient."

Despite these pathologic cautionary findings and the prevailing dogma of the Halsted Radical Mastectomy for 50 years or more, pioneering surgeons advocated less radical operations.

In 1943, Adair [31] reported his series of 63 patients with operable mammary cancer treated by local excision. Twenty-nine patients had conservative surgery followed by radiation therapy and experienced a 72% 5-year survival rate. Twenty-seven women had preoperative radiation therapy followed by local excision with a 70% 5-year survival, whereas seven patients had only local excision and six survived at the 5-year level.

Mustakallio [32], reporting from the Central Institute of Radiotherapy in Helsinki, described 127 patients treated by breast conserving surgery and radiation therapy. Several perceptive observations were made in this early publication. "I thus arrived at the conclusion that extirpation of the tumour, sparing the breast, and roentgen treatment is a satisfactory method in those cases of breast cancer in which lymph-nodes cannot be palpated in the axilla or the supraclavicular fossa and in which the primary tumor is not larger than a hen's egg. The removal of the tumour must, of course, be performed by careful dissection, leaving only sound tissue. According to my estimate, one-third of all cases of breast cancer arriving for treatment can be considered suitable for this treatment. I do not believe that it will be long before half the breast cancer patients present themselves for treatment early enough to be treated in the conservative way indicated above." Today 60% to 80% of patients with stage 0, I, and II are considered candidates for breast-conserving treatment.

Although Mustakallio's results were comparable to more radical surgery, others were reporting failures in breast-conserving surgery. Patey's classical 1948 description of modified radical mastectomy [17] included 10 cases in which partial mastectomy was combined with removal of the pectoralis minor muscle, full axillary dissection, and postoperative radiation therapy. Although these patients did as well as those undergoing more radical surgery, 20% recurred locally. Patey abandoned this procedure and concluded "that while in an occasional case, partial mastectomy combined with a dissection of the axilla might be justifiable, the danger of further development of carcinoma in the remaining breast tissue renders the procedure an unwise routine."

Significant negativism toward breast conservation occurred following the reports of unfavorable outcomes from the first randomized clinical trial comparing breast-conserving surgery to radical mastectomy. This trial was initiated by Sir Hedley Atkins at the Guy's Hospital in 1961 [33]. Three hundred seventy-four patients with operable breast cancer were randomized to either radical mastectomy and postoperative radiotherapy or wide excision, no axillary surgery, and postoperative irradiation. Both groups received 25 to 27 Gy to the axilla. The breast-conserving group received 35 to 38 Gy to the breast. The 10-year results revealed a significantly increased risk for local or regional recurrence in the wide excision group (25% versus 7%); however, only three patients out of a total of 45 with local-regional recurrence had in-breast recurrence. The majority of recurrences, as expected, occurred in the axilla, which had not been treated surgically, and was treated inadequately with radiation therapy. There was no significant difference in overall survival for stage I patients, but patients with stage II disease treated by wide excision experienced a 60% morality rate versus 30% for the radical mastectomy group. At this point trial entry was closed to women with stage II disease.

A second trial at Guy's Hospital accrued 258 patients with clinical stage I disease between 1971 and 1975 and reported by Hayward [34]. Using the same treatment arms, local-regional recurrence was reported in 30% of the breast conserving group versus 8% of the radical mastectomy group after a mean follow-up of 9 years. In addition, a significant difference was observed in mortality. Sixty percent of breast-conserving patients survived versus 82% of radical mastectomy patients.

As Fentiman [35] pointed out, one of the most significant findings in this study related to the increased risk for mortality in the conservatively treated group. This ran directly contrary to the prevailing thought that the form of local treatment had no impact on prognosis. This 25-year follow-up report continued to demonstrate that inadequate treatment of the axilla led to higher regional recurrences and increased mortality.

These results did not dissuade several surgical investigators from pursuing nonrandomized studies on breast-conserving surgery. In 1964, Porritt [36] reported 5- and 10-year follow-ups on 263 patients treated with segmental mastectomy and postoperative radiation therapy in most patients. Axillary lymph nodes were removed only if palpable. No comment was made about evaluation of segmental mastectomy margins. Survival rates were comparable to patients undergoing radical mastectomy. No data were reported on local recurrence. Porritt concluded that "without decreasing survival rates, a simple method of treatment has been employed which has eliminated deformity and reduced morbidity."

George Crile, Jr., from the Cleveland Clinic, is widely recognized as a pioneer in local excision for breast cancer. His initial report appeared in the *American Journal of Surgery* in 1965, and involved 20 patients selected between 1955 and 1958 to undergo quadrantectomy [37]. The average size in clinically node negative patients was 2.45 cm and 3.1 cm in patients with clinically suspicious axillary nodes. Five-year survival rates were equivalent to those undergoing mastectomy. Local recurrence was observed in one patient out of 12 with clinical stage I disease and four of eight in stage II disease. Dr. Crile was careful in his discussion in this manuscript to advocate a highly selective process for breast conserving surgery, stating that he "does not recommend that breast tumors be treated routinely or even commonly by local excision."

Crile's results were reported again in 1971 and included 55 patients undergoing quadrantectomy. In some cases he reported hemimastectomy for lower hemisphere lesions. This study confirmed earlier observations regarding survival equivalence with more radical surgery. Despite the fact that only three patients out of 40 with clinical stage I cancer undergoing breast-conserving surgery had postoperative radiation therapy, the 5-year local recurrence rate was only 5%. When stage I and stage II patients were included the local recurrence was 11% after quadrantectomy and 8% after mastectomy. Crile alluded to the need for randomized clinical trials in this manuscript observing that "If a study could be made in which treatment of small peripherally located carcinomas was randomized between local excision and mastectomy and if this study showed little, or no, difference in the incidence of locally recurrent tumors or in the survival rate, women could be assured that small carcinomas of the breast could be treated without loss of the breast" [38].

By 1985, the Cleveland Clinic had accumulated a series of 291 patients with breast-conserving surgery as reported by Hermann [21]. This represented 18% of 1593 patients with breast cancer treated between 1957 and 1975. Partial mastectomy without radiation therapy provided 5 to 15 years survival rates equal to modified radical mastectomy and total mastectomy. Local in-breast recurrence in the conservative group was observed to be 11% at 5 years, 15% at 10 years, and 16% at 15 years. Local recurrence was equivalent in the patients treated by mastectomy.

Vera Peters [39], from the Princess Margaret Hospital in Toronto, is also widely regarded as an early advocate of the conservative management of breast cancer. Between 1939 and 1972, 19 patients underwent excision alone and 184 underwent excision plus radiation therapy for a total of 203 versus 57 patients with mastectomy and 552 with mastectomy plus radiation therapy for a total of 609 patients. No significant differences were observed in survival rates or local recurrence.

Numerous nonrandomized studies of breast-conserving surgery and radiation therapy have appeared in the medical literature [40–57]. All of these studies, recognizing the flaws in nonrandomized studies such as selection bias, demonstrated encouraging outcomes for local control and survival using a combination of conservative breast surgery and radiation therapy.

Randomized clinical trials

The concept of a randomized clinical trial to minimize bias and assess the efficacy of one treatment versus another began in Europe over 50 years ago, and is now widely accepted as a gold standard for providing level I evidence

Table 3
Prospective randomized trials comparing conservative surgery and radiation with mastectomy for early-stage breast cancer

Trial	Treatment period	Total number of patients	Stage	Surgery for primary	Adjuvant therapy
Milan I	1973–1980	701	I	Q,RM	CMF
Instut Gustav-Roussy	1972–1980	179	I	WE,MRM	None
NSABP B-06	1976–1984	1219	I-II	WE,MRM	Melphalan, 5FU
NCI	1979–1987	237	I-II	WE,MRM	AC
EORTC	1980–1986	868	I-II	LE,MRM	CMF
Danish Breast Cancer Group	1983–1989	904	I-III	Q,WE, MRM	CMF Tamoxifen

Abbreviations: 5-FU, 5-fluorouracil; AC, Doxorubicin, Cyclophosphamide; CMF, Cyclophosphamide, Methotrexate, 5-fluorouracil; EORTC, European Organization for Research and Treatment of Cancer; LE, Local excision; MRM, modified radical mastectomy; Q, quadrantectomy; RM, radical mastectomy; WE, wide excision.

Reproduced with permission *from* Marrow M, Strom EA, Bassett LW, et al. Standard for breast conservation therapy in the management of invasive breast cancer. Ca Cancer J Clin 2002;52(5);278.

Table 4
Survival comparisons for conservative surgery and radiation (CS and RT) versus mastectomy in prospective randomized trials

Trial	Endpoint	Overall survival % CS and RT/mastectomy	Disease-free survival % CS and RT/mastectomy
Milan I	18 years	65 (NS) 65	
Institut			
Gustave-Roussy	15 years	73 (.19) 65	
NSABP B-06	12 years	63 (.12) 59	50 (.21) 49
NCI	10 years	77 (.89) 75	72 (.93) 69
EORTC	10 years	65 (NS) 66	
Danish Breast			
Cancer Group	6 years	79 (NS) 82	70 (NS) 66

Abbreviations: ( ), *P* value; EORTC, European Organization for Research and Treatment of Cancer; NS, not significant.

Reproduced with permission *from* Morrow M, Strom EA, Bassett LW, et al. Standard for breast conservation therapy in the management of invasive breast cancer. Ca Cancer J Clin 2002;52(5);279.

[58]. Eleven years elapsed between the 1961 Guy's Hospital randomized trial and six major, more contemporary randomized trials initiated between 1972 and 1983 [59–64]. The results summarized in Tables 3, 4, and 5, describe the trial design, survival comparisons, and local recurrence comparisons. Two of these six trials [62,63] reported a statistically significant increase in local recurrence in the conservative surgery and radiation therapy arm versus mastectomy. However, the National Cancer Institute trial [62] required only gross tumor removal without verification of microscopically free margins.

Table 5
Comparisons of local recurrence following conservative surgery and radiation (CS and RT) or mastectomy in prospective randomized trials

Trial	Endpoint	CS and RT	Mastectomy
Milan I	Cumulative incidence at 18 years	7% (NS)	4%
Institut			
Gustave-Roussy	Cumulative incidence at 15 years	9% (NS)	14%
NSABP B-06	Cumulative Incidence	10%	8%
NCI	Crude incidence median follow-up at 10.1 years	19% (.01)	6%
EORTC	Actuarial at 10 years	20% (.01)	12%
Danish Breast			
Cancer Group	Crude incidence median follow-up at 3.3 years	3% (NS)	4%

Abbreviations: ( ), *P* value; EORTIC, European Organization for Research and Treatment of Cancer; NS, not significant.

Reproduced with permission *from* Morrow M, Strom EA, Bassett LW, et al. Standard for breast conservation therapy in the management of invasive breast cancer. Ca Cancer J Clin 2002;52(5);280.

The European Organization for Research and Treatment of Cancer Trial [63] reported that 48% of patients in the breast-conserving arm had microscopically positive margins.

In 2002, *A Standard for Breast Conservation Therapy in the Management of Invasive Breast Carcinoma* was updated from a previous standard involving representatives from the American College of Radiology, the American College of Surgeons, the College of American Pathology, and the Society of Surgical Oncology [65]. Taking into account varying levels of evidence, this multidisciplinary group agreed on absolute and relative contraindications for breast conservation surgery and radiation therapy (Boxes 1 and 2).

From evidence to action: tracking national patterns of care

It is well known that many years elapse between level I evidence-based treatment recommendations and implementation at the point of care [66]. One method of communicating treatment practice change to the medical profession is through National Institutes of Health Consensus Conferences. Such a conference was convened by the National Institutes of Health on the treatment of early-stage breast cancer [67]. One of the major conclusions from that panel was "Breast conservation treatment is an appropriate

---

Box 1. Absolute contraindications

1. Pregnancy is an absolute contraindication to the use of breast irradiation. However, in many cases, it may be possible to perform breast-conserving surgery in the third trimester and treat the patient with irradiation after delivery.
2. Women with two or more primary tumors in separate quadrants of the breast or with diffuse malignant-appearing microcalcifications are not considered candidates for breast conservation treatment.
3. A history of prior therapeutic irradiation to the breast region that would require retreatment to an excessively high total-radiation dose to a significant volume is another absolute contraindication.
4. Persistent positive margins after reasonable surgical attempts. The importance of a single focally positive microscopic margin needs further study and may not be an absolute contraindication.

Adapted from Morrow M, Strom EA, Bassett LW, et al. Standard for breast conservation therapy in the management of invasive breast cancer. Ca Cancer J Clin 2002;52(5);289; with permission.

Box 2. Relative contraindications

1. A history of collagen vascular disease is a relative contraindication to breast conservation treatment because published reports indicate that such patients tolerate irradiation poorly. (*From* Fleck R, McNeese MD, Ellerbrock NA. Consequences of breast irradiation in patients with preexisting collagen vascular disease. Int J Radiat Oncol Biol Phys 1989;17:829–33, and Robertson JH, Clarke DH, Pevzner MM, et al. Breast conservation therapy: severe breast fibrosis after radiation therapy in patients with collagen vascular disease. Cancer 1991;68:501–8). Most radiation oncologists will not treat patients with scleroderma or active lupus erythematosus, considering it an absolute contraindication. In contrast, rheumatoid arthritis is not a relative or an absolute contraindication.

2. The presence of multiple gross tumors in the same quadrant and indeterminate calcifications must be carefully assessed for suitability because studies in this area are not definitive.

3. Tumor size is not an absolute contraindication to breast conservation treatment, although there is little published experience in treating patients with tumor sizes greater than 4 to 5 cm. However, a relative contraindication is the presence of a large tumor in a small breast in which an adequate resection would result in significant cosmetic alteration. In this circumstance, preoperative chemotherapy should be considered.

4. Breast size can be a relative contraindication. Treatment by irradiation of women with large or pendulous breasts is feasible if reproducibility of patient setup can be assured, and the technical capability exists for greater than or equal to six MV photon beam irradiation to obtain adequate dose homogeneity.

Adapted from Morrow M, Strom EA, Bassett LW, et al. Standard for breast conservation therapy in the management of invasive breast cancer. Ca Cancer J Clin 2002;52(5);289; with permission.

---

method of primary therapy for the majority of women with stage I and II breast cancer and is preferable because it provides survival rates equivalent to those of total mastectomy and axillary dissection while preserving the breast." A 1992 study from the National Cancer Database [68] described marked regional geographic variations in the use of breast-conserving treatment for early-stage breast cancer. This ranged from as low as 20% in some parts of the country to as high as 70% to 80% in other regions. Ten years later, in 2002, information from the National Cancer Database indicates that those regional variations have practically disappeared (A. Stewart, personal communication, National Cancer Database, American College of Surgeons, 2004).

In today's world serious attention must be devoted to evidence-based guidelines and continuous quality improvement of the cancer patient. The lessons learned from prospective randomized clinical trials need to be implemented in a more timely fashion for those caring for the cancer patient.

References

[1] Fabry W. Observationum et curationum chirurgicarum centuriae. I.A. Huguetan; 1641. p. 267–9.

[2] Brown J. Horae subsecivae. 2nd series. London: Adam & Charles Black; 1910. p. 277–8.

[3] Billroth T. General surgical pathology and therapeutics. New York: Appleton & Company; 1871. p. 658.

[4] Pancoast J. Treatise on operative surgery. Philadephia: Carey & Hart; 1844. p. 268.

[5] Halsted WS. The results of operations for the cure of cancer of the breast performed at the Johns Hopkins Hospital from June 1889 to January 1894. Johns Hopkins Hospital Rep 1894–1894:4:297–310.

[6] Harvey AM. Early contributions to the surgery of cancer: Halsted WS, Young HH, Clark JG. Hopkins Med J 1974;135:399–417.

[7] Taylor GW, Wallace RH. Carcinoma of the breast: fifty year's experience at the Massachusetts General Hospital. Ann Surg 1950;132(4):833–43.

[8] Handley WS. Parasternal invasion of the thorax in breast cancer and its suppression by the use of radium tubes as an operative precaution. Surg Gynecol Obstet 1927;45:721–8.

[9] Neuhof H. Excision of axillary vein in the radical operation for carcinoma of the breast. Ann Surg 1938;108:15–20.

[10] Gardner CE, McSwain GH, Moody JD. Removal of internal mammary lymphatics in carcinoma of the breast (preliminary report) [abstr]. Surgery 1951;30:270.

[11] Urban JA, Baker HW. Radical mastectomy in continuity with en bloc resection of the internal mammary lymph-node chain: a new procedure for primary operable cancer of the breast. Cancer 1952;5:992–1008.

[12] Haagensen CD, Stout AP. Carcinoma of the breast II. Criteria of operability. Ann Surg 1943;118:859 [continued on 1032].

[13] Baclesse F. La roentgentherapie seule dans le traitement des cancers du sein operables et inoperables. Troisieme rapport. Presented at the Association Francaise de Chirurgie, 51st Congress Francais de Chirurgie, Paris; 1948.

[14] Baclesse F. Roentgen therapy alone in cancer of the breast. Acta Un Int Cancer 1959;15: 1023.

[15] Murphy JB. Carcinoma of the breast. Surg Clin 1912;1(6):779.

[16] Grace E. Simple mastectomy in cancer of the breast. Am J Surg 1937;35:512.

[17] Patey DH, Dyson WH. The prognosis of carcinoma of the breast in relation to the type of operation performed. Br J Cancer 1927;2:7–13.

[18] Patey DH. A review of 146 cases of carcinoma of the breast operated on between 1930 and 1943. Br J Cancer 1967;21:260–9.

[19] Auchincloss H. Significance of location and number of axillary metastases in carcinoma of the breast. Ann Surg 1963;158:37–46.

[20] Madden JL. Modified radical mastectomy. Surg Gynecol Obstet 1965;121(6):1221–30.

[21] Hermann RE, Esselstyn CB Jr, Crile G Jr, et al. Results of conservative operations for breast cancer. Arch Surg 1985;120:746–51.

[22] Robinson GN, Van Heerden JA, Payne WS, et al. The primary surgical treatment of carcinoma of the breast: a changing trend toward modified radical mastectomy. Mayo Clin Proc 1976;51:433–42.

[23] Wilson RE, Donegan WL, Mettlin C, et al. The 1982 National Survey of Carcinoma of the Breast in the United States by the American College of Surgeons. Surg Gynecol Obstet 1984; 159:309–18.

[24] Turner L, Swindell R, Bell WGT, et al. Radical vs modified radical mastectomy for breast cancer. Ann R Coll Surg Engl 1981;63:239–43.

[25] Maddox WA, Carpenter JT Jr, Laws HL, et al. A randomized prospective trial of radical (Halsted) mastectomy versus modified radical mastectomy in 311 breast cancer patients. Ann Surg 1983;198(2):207–12.

[26] Fisher B, Redmond C, Fisher ER, et al. Ten-year results of a randomized clinical trial comparing radical mastectomy and total mastectomy with or without radiation. N Engl J Med 1985;312(11):674–81.

[27] Lewison EF. The surgical treatment of breast cancer; an historical and collective review. Surgery 1953;34(5):904–53.

[28] Gallager HS, Martin JE. Early phases in the development of breast cancer. Cancer 1969; 24(6):1170–8.

[29] Qualheim RE, Gall EA. Breast carcinoma with multiple sites of origin. Cancer 1957;10: 460–8.

[30] Schwartz GF, Patchesfsky AS, Feig SA, et al. Multicentricity of non-palpable breast cancer. Cancer 1980;45:2913–6.

[31] Adair FE. Role of surgery and irradiation in cancer of breast. JAMA 1943;121:553.

[32] Mustakallio S. Treatment of breast cancer by tumour extirpation and Roentgen therapy instead of radical operation. J Fac Rad 1954;6:23–6.

[33] Atkins HJB, Hayward JL, Klugman DJ, et al. Treatment of early breast cancer: a report after ten years of a clinical trial. BMJ 1972;2:423–9.

[34] Hayward JL. The Guy's Hospital trials on breast conservation. In: Harris JR, Hellman S, Silen W, editors. Conservative management of breast cancer. Philadelphia: J.B. Lippincott; 1983. p. 77–90.

[35] Fentiman IS. Long-term follow-up of the first breast conservation trial: Guy's wide excision study. Breast 2000;9:5–8.

[36] Porritt A. Early carcinoma of the breast. Br J Surg 1964;51:214–6.

[37] Crile G Jr. Treatment of breast cancer by local excision. Am J Surg 1965;109:400–3.

[38] Crile G Jr, Hoerr SO. Results of treatment of carcinoma of the breast by local excision. Surg Gynecol Obstet 1971;132:780–2.

[39] Peters MV. Wedge resection with or without radiation in early breast cancer. Int J Radiat Oncol Biol Phys 1977;11–12:1151–6.

[40] Fowble B, Solin LJ, Schultz DJ. Conservative surgery and radiation for early breast cancer. In: Fowble B, Goodman RL, Glick JH, Rosato EF, editors. Breast cancer treatment: a comprehensive guide to management. St. Louis (MO): Mosby Year Book; 1991. p. 105–50.

[41] Haffty BG, Goldberg NB, Rose M, et al. Conservative surgery with radiation therapy in clinical stage I and II breast cancer: Results of a 20-year experience. Arch Surg 1989;124: 1266–70.

[42] Leung S, Otmezguine Y, Calitchi E, et al. Locoregional recurrences following radical external beam irradiation and interstitial implantation for operable breast cancer: a twenty-three-year experience. Radiother Oncol 1986;5:1–10.

[43] Mansfield CM, Komarnicky LT, Schwartz GF, et al. Ten-year results in 1,070 patients with Stages I and II breast cancer treated by conservative surgery and radiation therapy. Cancer 1995;75:2328–36.

[44] Spitalier JM, Gambarelli J, Brandone H, et al. Breast-conserving surgery with radiation therapy for operable mammary carcinoma: a 25-year experience. World J Surg 1986;10: 1014–20.

[45] Stotter AT, McNeese MD, Ames FC, et al. Predicting the rate and extent of locoregional failure after breast conservation therapy for early breast cancer. Cancer 1989;64:2217–25.

[46] Kini VR, White JR, Horwitz EM, et al. Long-term results with breast-conserving therapy for patients with early stage breast carcinoma in a community hospital setting. Cancer 1998;82: 127–33.

[47] Dewar JA, Arriagada R, Benhamou S, et al. Local relapse and contralateral tumor rates in patients with breast cancer treated with conservative surgery and radiation therapy (Institut Gustave-Roussy 1970–1982). Cancer 1995;76:2260–5.

[48] Perez CA, Taylor ME, Halverson K, et al. Brachytherapy or electron beam boost in conservation therapy of carcinoma of the breast: a non-randomized comparison. Int J Radiat Oncol Biol Phys 1996;34:995–1007.

[49] Zafrani B, Vielh P, Fourquet A, et al. Conservative treatment of early breast cancer: prognostic value of the ductal in situ component and other pathological variables on local control and survival: long-term results. Eur J Cancer Clin Oncol 1989;25:1645–50.

[50] Gage I, Recht A, Gelman R, et al. Long-term outcome following breast-conserving surgery and radiation therapy. Int J Radiat Oncol Biol Phys 1995;33:245–51.

[51] Kurtz JM, Amalric R, Brandone H, et al. Local recurrence after breast-conserving surgery and radiotherapy: frequency, time course, and prognosis. Cancer 1989;63:1912–7.

[52] Kurtz JM, Amalric R, Delouche G, et al. The second ten-years: long-term risks of breast conservation in early breast cancer. Int J Radiat Oncol Biol Phys 1987;13:1327–32.

[53] Meric F, Mirza NQ, Valastos G, et al. Breast conservation surgery: long-term results from a single institution. Breast Cancer Res Treat 1999;57:51.

[54] Clark RM, Wilkinson RH, Mahoney LJ, et al. Breast cancer: a 21-year experience with conservative surgery and radiation. Int J Radiat Oncol Biol Phys 1982;8:967–79.

[55] Fowble B, Solin LJ, Schultz DJ, et al. Ten-year results of conservative surgery and radiation for stage I and II breast cancer. Int J Radiat Oncol Biol Phys 1991;21:269–77.

[56] Fourquet A, Campana F, Zafrani B, et al. Prognostic factors in the conservative management of early breast cancer: a 25-year follow-up at the Institute Curie. Int J Radiat Oncol Biol Phys 1989;17:719–25.

[57] Halverson KJ, Perez CA, Taylor ME, et al. Age is a prognostic factor for breast and regional node recurrence following breast conserving surgery and irradiation in Stage I and II breast cancer. Int J Radiat Oncol Biol Phys 1993;27:1045–50.

[58] Donegan WL. An introduction to the history of breast cancer. In: Donegan WL, Spratt JS, editors. Cancer of the breast. 5th edition. Philadelphia: WB Saunders; 2002. p. 1–15.

[59] Veronesi U, Banfi A, Del Vecchio M, et al. Comparison of Halsted mastectomy with quadrantectomy, axillary dissection and radiotherapy in early breast cancer: Long-term results. Eur J Cancer Clin Oncol 1986;22:1085–9.

[60] Arriagada R, Le MG, Rochard F, et al. Conservative treatment versus mastectomy in early breast cancer: patterns of failure in 15-years of follow-up data. Institut Gustave-Roussy Breast Cancer Group. J Clin Oncol 1996;14:1558–64.

[61] Fisher B, Redmond C, Poisson R, et al. Eight-year results of a randomized clinical trial comparing total mastectomy and lumpectomy with or without irradiation in the treatment of breast cancer. N Engl J Med 1989;320:822–8.

[62] Jacobson JA, Danforth DN, Cowan KH, et al. Ten-year results of a comparison of conservation with mastectomy in the treatment of stage I and II breast cancer. N Engl J Med 1995;332:907–11.

[63] Van Dongen JA, Bartelink H, Fentiman IS, et al. Factors influencing local relapse and survival and results of salvage treatment after breast-conserving therapy in operable breast cancer: EORTC trail 10801, breast conservation compared with mastectomy in TNM Stage I and II breast cancer. Eur J Cancer 1992;28A:801–5.

[64] Blichert-Toft M, Rose C, Anderson JA, et al. Danish randomized trial comparing breast conservation therapy with mastectomy: six-years of life-table analysis. Danish Breast Cancer Cooperative Group. J Natl Cancer Inst Monogr 1992;11:19–25.

[65] Morrow M, Strom EA, Bassett LW, et al. Standard for breast conservation therapy in the management of invasive breast cancer. CA Cancer J Clin 2002;52:277–300.

[66] Sung NS, Crowley WF Jr, Genel M, et al. Central challenges facing the national clinical research enterprise. JAMA 2003;289(10):1278–87.

[67] Treatment of early-stage breast cancer. NIH Consensus Conference. JAMA 1991;265(3): 391–5.

[68] Osteen RT, Steele GD, Menck HR, et al. Regional differences in the management of breast cancer. CA J Clin 1992;42:39–43.

ELSEVIER
SAUNDERS

Surg Oncol Clin N Am
14 (2005) 499–509

SURGICAL
ONCOLOGY CLINICS
OF NORTH AMERICA

Radical Lobectomy, Esophagectomy, and Mediastinal Dissections for Intrathoracic Malignancy

John C. Kucharczuk, MD[a], Larry R. Kaiser, MD[b],*

[a]Section of Thoracic Surgery, University of Pennsylvania School of Medicine,
3400 Spruce Street, 4 Silverstein Pavilion, Philadelphia, PA 19104-4227, USA
[b]Department of Surgery, University of Pennsylvania School of Medicine,
3400 Spruce Street, 4 Silverstein Pavilion, Philadelphia, PA 19104-4227, USA

In many ways, development of the radical resection of intrathoracic malignancies has paralleled developments in the surgical treatment of breast cancer. Early operations were aggressive, debilitating, and were associated with significant morbidity and mortality. Success with malignant disease seemed to be predicated on making the biggest possible operation, seemingly without regard for the fact that cancer is a systemic disease, with rare exception. There is no question that some patients were cured, based on control of the primary tumor, with an operation that left no doubt that all gross disease had been removed. The term "radical" can be interpreted in a number of ways. Removing all surrounding tissue, well beyond the primary tumor, could be thought of as radical with certain malignancies, whereas with other cancers, the complete removal of the regional lymph nodes qualifies an operation as radical. Halsted's landmark report on patients undergoing radical mastectomy demonstrated the value of radical resection for breast cancer [1]. He reported a reduction in the local recurrence rate of 50% better than the results achieved by his contemporaries in the United States and in Europe, as significant improvement over conventional approaches of the time. With time, however, Halsted's operation, like many other radical procedures, evolved into a less aggressive operation, the modified radical mastectomy, and now, with the addition of early screening studies and the application of multimodality treatments, lumpectomy with sentinel node sampling.

---

* Corresponding author.
E-mail address: kaiser@uphs.upenn.edu (L.R. Kaiser).

This evolution occurred primarily in response to our increasing knowledge of the biology of cancer and the recognition that we are dealing with a systemic disease that requires more than just control of the local disease to effect a cure. Much of our thinking regarding so-called radical operations for cancer stems from the efforts, in the mid-twentieth century, of the group of individuals assembled at what was then known as the Memorial Hospital for Cancer and Allied Diseases, now the Memorial Sloan-Kettering Cancer Center in New York City. This was the first hospital in the United States dedicated to the care and treatment of patients with malignant disease. Much of the early progress made at the hospital was driven by the pathologist James Ewing. Other individuals who contributed to the concept of radical surgery for cancer included Alexander Brunschwig (radical pelvic surgery), Hayes Martin (head and neck surgery), George Pack, Jerome Urban, and others.

Similarly, the treatment of lung cancer has passed from an era in which pneumonectomy was considered the only appropriate operation to our current management that includes an anatomic resection, usually lobectomy, in addition to complete mediastinal lymph node dissection, and often includes postoperative adjuvant chemotherapy. With advanced surgical techniques that are widely available, a pneumonectomy is avoided routinely in most situations, while preserving optimal rates of local control and long-term survival.

In contrast, the surgical management of esophageal malignancies continues to evolve. There is little consensus or data regarding the optimal surgical management of esophageal cancer, but we have seen a tremendous increase in the number of cases of adenocarcinoma over the past 25 years. Squamous carcinoma of the esophagus now has become relatively rare in the United States. Several surgical approaches to esophagectomy exist, ranging from the transhiatal approach to the three-field esophagectomy with radical lymph node dissection. Each approach has its own outspoken opponents and proponents, but despite the rhetoric, several studies have shown equivalent outcomes among the multiple approaches. No clear winner has emerged, and thus there is no "standard" surgical approach for esophageal cancer. The "complete" esophageal surgeon must be facile with a range of operations to deal effectively with the patient with esophageal cancer because one operation does not fit all.

This article reviews the application of radical resections in the treatment of intrathoracic malignancies, including lung and esophageal cancers. We also demonstrate how early radical surgical resections have influenced and evolved into the current treatment of these diseases.

Radical operations for lung cancer

In February of 1933, Evart Graham at Barnes Hospital in St. Louis, MO, performed the first successful one-stage pneumonectomy with seven-rib thoracoplasty for lung cancer [2]. Although it is an aggressive procedure, the operation was not by definition radical in that the hilar structures were divided using the technique of mass ligation, and no mediastinal lymph nodes were removed. This involved placing a tourniquet around the hilum, cinching it down, and then suturing the vessels and bronchus. One does not need to use one's imagination to visualize the scene if the tourniquet around the hilum slipped off. His operation and report, however, were the seminal event that sparked significant progress in the surgical management of bronchogenic carcinoma, a disease that at the time was believed to be extremely rare but now accounts for the number one cause of cancer death in both men and women. Within months of Graham's first successful operation, William Rienhoff of Johns Hopkins University significantly advanced the field when he successfully performed a left pneumonectomy using hilar dissection with individual ligation of the hilar structures [3]. By the 1940s, the incidence of lung cancer was increasing, and total removal of the lung was believed to be the only procedure that could possibly result in a cure [4]. Certainly, pneumonectomy, especially when considered in the context in which we view lung cancer today, would have been considered a radical operation at the time of Graham and Reinhoff, whether or not lymph nodes were removed. Just the concept of operating for a cancer of the lung was perceived to be radical, although it was not referred to as such.

In 1945, the concept of the radical pneumonectomy began to evolve. Allison [5] described the intrapericardial pneumonectomy, which allowed for resection of centrally located tumors as well as those with involvement of the mediastinal lymph nodes. Ochsner and DeBakey [6] realized that knowledge about the routes of lymphatic spread could be incorporated into a rational surgical approach to lung cancer. Shortly thereafter, Cahan and colleagues [7] at Memorial Hospital in New York City defined the operation that they referred to as a radical pneumonectomy. This operation involved resection of the lung, in continuity with the regional lymph nodes located within the hilum and mediastinum taken en bloc. The en bloc concept was believed to be an important part of this procedure, based on the knowledge gleaned from the treatment of breast cancer.

The radical pneumonectomy was perceived by many as the ultimate treatment for lung cancer. An early report from Churchill and colleagues [8], however, suggested that local control and long-term survival in early stage lung cancer was possible with lobectomy. In 1956, the value of the radical pneumonectomy was questioned in a report from Watson [9]. He observed no change in 5-year survival rates when comparing the outcomes of pneumonectomy, radical pneumonectomy, and lobectomy. This was followed by a report from Johnson and colleagues [10] from the University of Pennsylvania, which further called into question the rationale of insisting on a radical pneumonectomy as the optimal and preferred treatment of lung cancer. Cahan, who had earlier defined radical pneumonectomy, subsequently stepped in to coin the term "radical lobectomy." His manuscript detailing this approach included a 17-page description for the technique of en bloc removal of the mediastinal lymph nodes and the associated lobe containing a bronchogenic carcinoma [11]. In 1969, he reported on 48 patients treated with this technique [12]. Although he stressed the en bloc removal of the regional lymph nodes, it is interesting to note that it was nearly 20 years later when a systematic map of the hilar and mediastinal lymph nodes was put forth [13]. In many respects, the systematic nodal map ushered in our current techniques of staging and surgical resection for patients with lung cancer. We now recognize that the removal of the mediastinal lymph nodes likely does not confer a therapeutic benefit in and of itself. What it does accomplish, however, is the optimal staging of the disease so that the surgeon, oncologist, and patient have a better idea of the prognosis and whether there would be any benefit to postoperative adjuvant treatment, specifically chemotherapy. The accuracy of surgical staging cannot be overestimated as we attempt to learn more about this disease, especially in the context of clinical trials. It is difficult to conceive of a lobectomy with mediastinal lymph node dissection as radical because it is today the standard operation performed for lung cancer. Unfortunately, it is still common to find patients who have undergone pulmonary resection without the benefit of mediastinal lymph node dissection, leaving us with little idea of the true pathologic stage for those patients. To meet the standard of care for a pulmonary resection, the operation should at least include complete mediastinal lymph node sampling if not nodal dissection, a procedure that adds perhaps 15 minutes to the length of the case.

At present, patients who are medically fit and have no clinical evidence of mediastinal lymph node involvement are offered surgical resection as the primary therapy for cure. Even in early stage disease, lobectomy is considered the gold standard and is associated with improved survival over sublobar resections [14], whether anatomic segmental resection or nonanatomic wedge resection. Patients with biopsy-confirmed disease, ipsilateral mediastinal nodal disease, are offered neoadjuvant chemotherapy with or without radiation therapy and are then considered for curative resection. The role and extent of mediastinal lymph node dissection remains a matter of debate. Currently, there is no standardization between lymph node sampling and complete lymph node dissection during the performance of lobectomy for lung cancer. A recent American College of Surgeons Oncology Group study Z0030 trial randomized patients to either lymph node sampling or to complete lymph node dissection during pulmonary resection. The trial met accrual targets in late 2004, and the results are forthcoming.

A significant recent advance in lung cancer treatment has been the recognition of the value of postresection chemotherapy in patients with completely resected early stage lung cancer [15]. As with breast cancer, the majority of patients with lung cancer who are resected for cure are now evaluated for and offered postoperative chemotherapy.

Thus, in many respects, the evolution of the treatment of lung cancer has paralleled the treatment of breast cancer. We have moved away from very aggressive, locally morbid operations to safer, less radical procedures with similar and even improved outcomes. Both diseases have benefited from the application of a multimodal approach, including aggressive preoperative staging and systemic treatment. Just as in breast cancer, accurate staging has contributed greatly to our knowledge of both the natural history and best treatment options for lung cancer.

Radical operations for esophageal cancer

Franz Torek [16] performed the first successful esophagectomy for esophageal cancer in 1913. The lesion was located in the thoracic esophagus and was approached at surgery by dividing the left diaphragm. Its removal required partial mobilization of the aorta and repair of the left main stem bronchus, which was torn during resection. A primary anastomosis was not performed because no methods had yet been described for using either the colon or the stomach for esophageal replacement. Gastrointestinal continuity was reestablished with the use of an external rubber tube, which connected a cervical esophagostomy to a gastrostomy. The tube could be removed for cleaning to keep it patent. Remarkably, the patient survived the operation and lived an additional 13 years. Nevertheless, esophageal resection remained a formidable undertaking, and no successful attempts were reported for another 20 years.

In 1933, Turner [17] reported the first transhiatal esophagectomy for cancer. The operation differed significantly from the modern transhiatal resection in that the patient's gastrointestinal continuity was reconstructed with a skin tube at a second stage, performed later. Five years later, Adams and Phemister reported on a successful left transpleural resection of a distal esophageal carcinoma with immediate reconstruction through an esophagogastrostomy, transposing a portion of the stomach into the chest. In 1945, Sweet [18] reported placing the esophagogastric anastomosis high in the left chest to resect midthoracic esophageal lesions. This procedure required complete mobilization of the gastric remnant, basing the blood supply on the right gastroepiploic vessels, truly a radical concept. Shortly thereafter, Ivor Lewis [19] proposed a two-hole operation, which involved a laparotomy for mobilization of the stomach and subsequently a right thoracotomy for resection of the esophagus and reconstruction and anastomosis within the chest. In 1962, McKeown [20] described the three-field esophagectomy, which included an upper abdominal incision, a right thoracotomy, and a left neck incision, with placement of the anastomosis in the cervical location. It was the combination of these major milestones in esophageal surgery over 30 years that set the stage for the radical esophagectomy popularized by Skinner in the 1980s. Each of the early procedures mentioned was truly radical for the time they were proposed and performed. To even imagine performing an esophagectomy in the pre-antibiotic era, when entry into the chest was essentially impossible, is truly a remarkable feat and one of considerable daring on the part of the patient and the surgeon.

Skinner, influenced by his surgical training under Sir Ronald Belsey at the Frenchay Hospital in Bristol, U.K. and an early report on the application of wide field regional lymph node dissection in the treatment of cancers of the cardia [21], described an operation to remove the esophagus with its surrounding lymph node basin. The operation was carefully standardized, and significant emphasis was placed on preoperative staging to select appropriate candidates for "curative" resections. The goal of the operation was a 10-cm axial margin with a complete radical lymph node dissection. The thoracic component of the operation aimed to remove an envelope of tissue surrounding the esophagus, which included: the mediastinal pleura, the azygos vein, the thoracic duct, the posterior pericardium, the mediastinal lymph nodes, and the intercostals arteries, truly a radical esophagectomy. In the neck, a U-shaped incision was made, and dissection included the supraclavicular and deep cervical lymph nodes as well as lymph nodes along the recurrent laryngeal nerves. Despite this aggressive dissection of the lymph nodes in the neck, the rate of recurrent nerve injury was reported as occurring only in 6% of the patients [22].

Skinner's [23] initial report detailed the results on a cohort of 80 patients who were treated by radical en bloc resection carcinomas involving the lower, middle, and upper esophagus. He concluded that radical en bloc resection for carcinoma of the esophagus could, in experienced hands, be performed with a mortality rate equivalent to a standard esophagectomy. In addition, he stressed the use of this radical operation to provide improved pathologic staging as a guide for prognosis and the consideration of postoperative adjuvant therapy. A small number of patients were long-term survivors, despite multiple seemingly unfavorable prognostic factors. Fifteen years latter, he was able to demonstrate improved survival in a highly selected cohort of patients with stage III disease who underwent radical en bloc resection compared with standard resection [24]. The updated study was a retrospective review of a prospectively established database but did show an improvement in 3-year survival rates from 13% for standard esophagectomy to 34% in patients undergoing radical resection.

Interestingly, during the same general time frame in which Skinner was promoting the radical esophagectomy, Orringer was re-introducing the transhiatal total esophagectomy, which had been described first by Turner in 1933. Orringer had perfected and refined the "esophagectomy without thoracotomy" and touted it as the standard operation for esophageal cancer, with the view that the procedure could be performed with significantly less morbidity and mortality because the chest was not entered. Regional lymph nodes could be taken through this approach and adequate staging performed. In contrast to Turner's second-stage skin tube reconstruction to reestablish gastrointestinal continuity, Orringer provided immediate reconstruction preferentially with a conduit fashioned from the gastric remnant and placed the anastomosis in the neck. Getting the gastric remnant to the neck could be accomplished in every case with complete mobilization of the stomach, including division of the short gastric vessels, the coronary vein, and left gastric artery, total mobilization of the greater curvature of the stomach, and a Kocher maneuver. The pylorus would be located at the hiatus when the stomach was transposed to the neck through the posterior mediastinum. Taking off a portion of the lesser curvature also allowed for additional length to allow the gastric remnant to reach the neck. Orringer presented his findings and technique at the 1978 meeting of the American Association for Thoracic Surgery in New Orleans, and he and Sloan subsequently published their experience with 26 patients [25]. They concluded that the operation was safe and better tolerated from a physiologic perspective than more traditional techniques used for esophageal resection and reconstruction. The ability to stay out of the chest added to the attractiveness of the procedure, with the thought being that there would be a decreased incidence of pulmonary complications. The popularization of this approach also led to a shift in thinking about the nature and extent of disease in patients with esophageal carcinoma. Again, as in the modern treatment of breast cancer and more recently lung cancer, the concept of esophageal cancer as a systemic rather than a localized disease emerged. Orringer conceived of resection in patients with esophageal cancer as part of a multimodal treatment plan. He pointed to his University of Michigan esophageal cancer protocol, which included 43 patients with esophageal carcinomas treated with preoperative chemotherapy (cisplatin, vinblastine, and fluorouracil) and concurrent radiation therapy followed by transhiatal esophagectomy. The 2-year survival rate in these patients improved to 59% compared with 30% in those treated by resection alone [26]. Interestingly, further support for Orringer's concept was provided by a report by Altorki and Skinner [22] in 1997 on occult cervical nodal metastasis in thoracic esophageal cancer. They found 35% of patients had occult cervical nodal metastasis irrespective of the tumor location and suggested these data supported the concept of very aggressive three-field nodal dissection for esophageal cancer, what they referred to as their radical esophagectomy. In an editorial, however, Orringer argued that their data supported the concept of esophageal cancer as a systemic disease that was unlikely to be cured by surgery alone [27]. He posed the pertinent question, "where does the lymph node chase end?" Both sides suggested further investigation was warranted to determine the optimal surgical approach to esophageal cancer, a view that still exists today, despite the emergence of the radical operation.

Currently, the debate regarding the extent of resection in esophageal cancer continues. A contemporary randomized trial from the Netherlands comparing transhiatal resection with transthoracic resection with en bloc lymphadenectomy (the more radical procedure) failed to show a statistically significant survival advantage of one technique of the other [28]. There was, however, a 30% higher rate of pulmonary complications in the radical transthoracic group compared with patients undergoing transhiatal resection.

The role of combined modality treatment also remains undetermined. A number of randomized trials have failed to show any benefit from preoperative radiation therapy alone. A meta-analysis of available randomized trials comprising 1147 patients found no improvement in survival with preoperative radiotherapy alone in patients with resectable esophageal cancer [29]. At this time there is no indication for preoperative radiation therapy alone followed by resection.

The value of preoperative chemotherapy alone is much more poorly defined. A large multicentered randomized trial in the United States (Intergroup Trial) [30] of 440 patients failed to show any improvement in survival after three cycles of combined cisplatin and fluorouracil followed by surgery and two postoperative cycles when compared with surgery alone. This is in contrast to a large randomized European study (Medical Research Council) [31], which suggested that neoadjuvant chemotherapy resulted in a nearly 10% improvement in survival at 2 years. Unfortunately, the preoperative staging techniques and treatment durations were quite different, making the two studies difficult to compare. From an evidence-based perspective, a recent review of 11 randomized controlled trials with 2051 patients has suggested that there was improved survival in patients who underwent preoperative chemotherapy followed by resection; however, it did not reach statistical significance until 5 years, and there was increased toxicity and mortality in the chemotherapy group [32]. This issue remains unresolved and operation remains the standard treatment for esophageal cancer outside of a clinical trial.

There have been several small randomized trials evaluating combined preoperative chemo-radiation therapy followed by surgical resection. The most widely cited trial, which is often used to justify combined modality treatment followed by surgery, was published by Walsh and colleagues in 1996 [33]. This study projected a 3-year survival rate of 32% in the neoadjuvant treatment group compared with 6% in the surgery alone group for patients with adenocarcinoma. Critics are quick to point out the lack of appropriate standardized staging, the poor survival in the surgical group compared with other surgical series, and the small study size. A more recent study found an equivalent median and 3-year survival rate in patients with squamous cell carcinoma of the esophagus who were randomized to either preoperative chemo-radiation therapy followed by surgery versus surgery alone [34]. An increased complication rate was noted in the patients undergoing preoperative chemo-radiation therapy. Unfortunately, a large cooperative group trial involving several of the larger cooperative groups designed to answer this question was forced to close because of poor accrual. There is still a tremendous bias that exists among physicians and patients alike that surgery is the treatment of choice and delaying operation to get in a few cycles of chemotherapy is not warranted, despite the fact that the question regarding preoperative therapy has yet to be answered. This bias makes it extremely difficult to enroll patients in a randomized trial in which surgery is involved.

Of the several surgical approaches to esophagectomy, each has its own set of risks and benefits as well as outspoken opponents and proponents. The selection of an appropriate approach for an individual patient requires experienced surgical judgment. Despite the rhetoric, several studies have shown equivalent outcomes among the multiple surgical approaches. It appears that the experience of the surgeon [35] and the volume of like cases performed at a particular institution are the most important factors determining outcome [36]. A recent high-volume, single-institution review has showed that technical complications following esophagectomy were associated with increased length of hospital stay and increased inhospital mortality and were predictive of a poorer overall long-term survival [37]. Whether more aggressive surgical resections or advances in multimodal treatments will improve outcomes in esophageal cancer remains to be seen. The goal of esophageal resection, whether it is used as the primary treatment or as part of a multimodality plan is cure; although this goal remains elusive. At present, "we need to continue to work toward reducing the rate of perioperative complications associated with esophagectomy and defining the variables that relate to long-term survival" [38].

Summary

In many respects, the evolution of the treatment of intrathoracic malignancies, including lung and esophageal cancer, has paralleled the experience with breast cancer. Initial operations were aggressive and highly morbid but did result in occasional long-term survival in an otherwise hopeless situation. With improvements in operative techniques and postoperative care, the mortality associated with resection began to fall. More recently, the concept of intrathoracic malignancies as systemic diseases has evolved. Multimodal approaches are becoming more common in the treatment of lung cancer. The optimal treatment of esophageal cancer still remains to be defined, but numerous investigators are working on the problem because the incidence of adenocarcinoma has increased so markedly.

References

[1] Halsted WS. The results of operations for cure of cancer of the breast from June 1889 to January 1894. Johns Hopkins Hospital Report 1894–1895;4:297.

[2] Graham EA, Singer JJ. Successful removal of an entire lung for carcinoma of the bronchus. JAMA 1933;101:1371–4.

[3] Reinhoff WF. A preliminary report of the operative technique in two successful cases. Bull Hist Med 1933;53:390.

[4] Graham EA. Indications for total pneumonectomy. Chest (Diseases of the Chest) 1944;10:87.

[5] Allision PR. Intrapericardial approach to the lung root in the treatment of bronchial carcinoma by dissection pneumonectomy. J Thorac Cardiovasc Surg (Journal of Thoracic Surgery) 1946;15:99.

[6] Ochsner A, DeBakey M. Significance of metastasis in primary carcinoma of the lung. J Thorac Cardiovasc Surg (Journal of Thoracic Surgery) 1942;11:357.

[7] Cahan WG, Watson WI, Pool JL. Radical pneumonectomy. J Thorac Cardiovasc Surg (Journal of Thoracic Surgery) 1951;22:449.

[8] Churchill ED, Sweet RH, Sutter L, et al. The surgical management of carcinoma of the lung: a study of cases treated at the Massachusetts General Hospital from 1930–1950. J Thorac Cardiovasc Surg 1950;20:349.

[9] Watson WL. Carcinoma of the lung with five-year survivals: a study of 3,000 cases. Cancer 1956;9:1167–72.

[10] Johnson J, Kirby CK, Blakemore WS. Should we insist on "radical pneumonectomy" as a routine procedure in the treatment of carcinoma of the lung? J Thorac Cardiovasc Surg (Journal of Thoracic Surgery) 1958;36:309–15.

[11] Cahan WG. Racial lobectomy. J Thorac Cardiovasc Surg 1960;39:555–72.

[12] Ramsey HE, Cahan WG, Deattie EJ, et al. The importance of radical lobectomy in lung cancer. J Thorac Cardiovasc Surg 1969;58(2):225–30.

[13] Naruke T, Suemasu K, Ishikawa S. Lymph node mapping and curability at various levels of metastasis in resected lung cancer. J Thorac Cardiovasc Surg 1978;76:832–9.

[14] Ginsberg RJ. The comparison of limited resection to lobectomy for T1No non-small cell lung cancer: LCSG 821. Chest 1994;106:3185–95.

[15] Strauss GM, Herndon J, Maddaus MA, et al. Randomized clinical trial of adjuvant chemotherapy with paclitaxel and carboplatin following resection in stage IB non-small cell lung cancer (NSCLC): report of Cancer and Leukemia Group B (CALGB) protocol 9633 [abstract]. J Clin Oncol 2004;22(Suppl 14) A-7019, S621.

[16] Torek F. The first successful case of resection of the thoracic portion of the esophagus for carcinoma. J Am Coll Surg (Surgery, Gynecology & Obstetrics) 1913;16:614–7.

[17] Turner GG. Excision of thoracic esophagus for carcinoma with construction of extra-thoracic gullet. Lancet 1933;2:1315.

[18] Sweet RH. Surgical management of carcinoma of the midthoracic esophagus: preliminary report. N Engl J Med 1945;233:1.

[19] Lewis I. The surgical treatment of carcinoma of the oesophagus with special reference to a new operation for growths of the middle third. Br J Surg 1946;34:18.

[20] McKeown K. Three stage oesphagectomy for cancer of the oesophagus. Br J Surg 1976;63:259.

[21] Logan A. The surgical treatment of carcinoma of the esophagus and cardia. J Thorac Cardiovasc Surg 1963;46:150.

[22] Altorki NK, Skinner DB. Occult cervical nodal metastasis in esophageal cancer: preliminary results of three-field lymphadenectomy. J Thorac Cardiovasc Surg 1997;113:540–4.

[23] Skinner DB. En bloc resection for neoplasms of the esophagus and cardia. J Thorac Cardiovasc Surg 1983;85:59.

[24] Altorki NK, Giradi L, Skinner DB. En bloc esophagectomy improves survival for stage III esophageal cancer. J Thorac Cardiovasc Surg 1997;114(6):948–55.

[25] Orringer MB, Sloan H. Esophagectomy without thoracotomy. J Thorac Cardiovasc Surg 1978;76(5):643–54.

[26] Orringer MD. Ten-year survival after esophagectomy for carcinoma: surgical triumph of biologic variation. Chest 1989;96(5):970.

[27] Altorki NK, Skinner DB. Occult cervical nodal metastatses in esophageal cancer: preliminary results of three-filed lymphadenectomy [editorial]. J Thorac Cardiovasc Surg 1997;113:538–9.
[28] Hullscher J, Van Sandick J, Van Lanschot J. Extended transthoracic resection compared with limited transhiatal resection for adenoxarcinoma of the esophagus. N Engl J Med 2002; 347:1662–9.
[29] Arnott SJ, Duncan W, Gignoux M, et al, for the Oeosphageal Cancer Collaborative Group. Preoperative radiotherapy for esophageal carcinoma. Cochrane Review 2004;4.
[30] Kelsen DP, Ginsberg RJ. Chemotherapy followed by surgery compared with surgery alone for localized esophageal cancer. N Engl J Med 1998;339:1979–84.
[31] Medical Research Council Oesophageal Cancer Working Group. Surgical resection with or without postoperative chemotherapy in oesophageal cancer: a randomised controlled trial. Lancet 2002;359:1727–33.
[32] Malthaner R, Fenlon D. Preoperative chemotherapy for resectable thoracic esophageal cancer. Cochrane Database Syst Rev 2003;4:CD001556.
[33] Walsh T, Noonan N, Hollywood D, et al. A comparison of multimodal therapy and surgery for esophageal adenocarcinoma. N Engl J Med 1996;335:462–7.
[34] Bosset J-F, Marc Gignoux M, Triboulet J-P, et al. Chemoradiotherapy followed by surgery compared with surgery alone in squamous-cell cancer of the esophagus. N Engl J Med 1997; 337(3):161–7.
[35] Bolten JS, Teng S. Transthoracic or transhiatal esophagectomy for cancer of the esophagus: does it matter? Surg Oncol Clin N Am 2002;11(2):365–75.
[36] Dimick JB, Pronovost PJ, Cowan JA, et al. Surgical volume and quality of care for esophageal resection: do high-volume hospitals have fewer complications? Ann Thorac Surg 2003;75(2):337–41.
[37] Rizk NP, Bach PB, Schrag D, et al. The impact of complications on outcomes after resection for esophageal and gastroesophageal junction carcinoma. J Am Coll Surg 2004;198:42–50.
[38] Kaiser LR. Is there a "standard of care" operation for esophageal cancer? [editorial]. Ann Surg 2001;235(5):588–9.

ELSEVIER
SAUNDERS

Surg Oncol Clin N Am
14 (2005) 511–532

SURGICAL
ONCOLOGY CLINICS
OF NORTH AMERICA

Radical Gastrectomy and Lymphadenectomy: Historic Overview, Surgical Trends, and Lessons from the Past

Michael R. DiSiena, DO[a], Charu Taneja, MD, FACS[a,b], Harold J. Wanebo, MD[b,c,d],*

[a]Department of Surgery, Roger Williams Medical Center, 825 Chalkstone Avenue, Providence, RI 02908, USA
[b]Department of Surgery, Boston University School of Medicine, 715 Albany Street, Boston, MA 02118, USA
[c]Department of Surgery, Brown University School of Medicine, Providence, RI 02912, USA
[d]Division of Surgical Oncology, Department of Surgery, Roger Williams Medical Center, 825 Chalkstone Avenue, Providence, RI 02908, USA

Epidemiology and trends in the incidence of gastric carcinoma

In the course of the past century, gastric cancer has been one of the most common causes of cancer-related mortality among American men and women in the pre-World War II era [1]. Since the early period of the twentieth century, the incidence of gastric cancer has declined sharply among American men and women (Fig. 1) [2].

The incidence of gastric cancer in the United States in 2003 was 22,400 diagnosed cases, and the mortality was reportedly 12,100 deaths [2]. Gastric cancer is now an infrequent cause of cancer-related deaths among American men and women [2]. The cause of this trend is not known completely, but perhaps changing environmental factors are contributing to the decline. While the incidence of distal gastric cancers has steadily declined since 1930, there has been an increase in the number of proximal gastric cancers in the American population, in contrast to the Japanese, in whom distal gastric cancers still are predominant [3–8]. The increased number of diagnosed

* Corresponding author.
E-mail address: hwanebo@RWMC.org (H.J. Wanebo).

1055-3207/05/$ - see front matter © 2005 Elsevier Inc. All rights reserved.
doi:10.1016/j.soc.2005.05.002

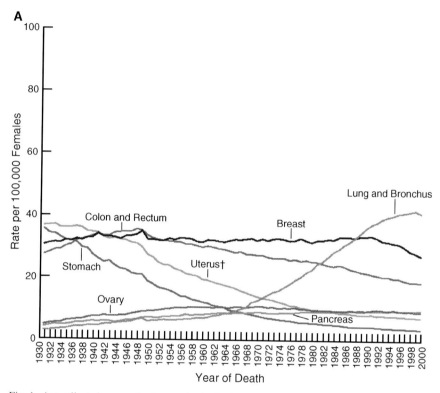

Fig. 1. Age-adjusted cancer death rates in the United States from 1930 to 2000 for women (*A*) and men (*B*), showing a declining death rate for gastric cancer. (*Data from* Jemal A, Murray T, Samuels A, et al. Cancer statistic 2003. CA Cancer J Clin 2003;53:5–26.)

proximal gastric cancers may be shadowed by the relative decline in the number of distal gastric cancers contributing to a relatively higher incidence of more frequently detected proximal cancers.

Extent of gastric resection

Early surgical history of gastric surgery for cancer

The first reported gastrectomies were attempted unsuccessfully by Pean (1875) and Rydigear (1880) for gastric cancer; both patients died in the immediate postoperative period [9–11]. The father of gastric surgery was Christian A.T. Billroth (1829–1894), a Viennese surgeon, who, on January 29, 1881, performed the first successful gastrectomy for cancer [12]. Billroth reported to Witelshofer, in a letter dated February 4, 1881, that he performed a pylorectomy with an end-to-end gastroduodenostomy [12,13]. The operation was successful, and his patient survived for 4 months until she

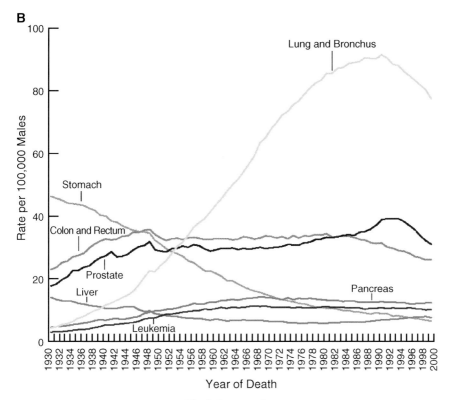

Fig. 1 (*continued*)

succumbed to disease progression and death [12]. Subsequently, Billroth reported a surgical variation that allowed for closure of the duodenal stump and the creation of a gastrojejunostomy, which was reported in 1885 [12]. During the course of Billroth's successful and productive career, he performed 34 gastrectomies for gastric cancer, over a 13-year period [12].

Several years later, in 1884, the first total gastrectomy for gastric cancer was attempted by Connor in Cincinnati, OH, and performed later by Schlatter (1897) in Switzerland [14]. Schlatter was given the credit for the first successful total gastrectomy because his patient survived the operation. The success of technical achievements by Billroth and Schlatter marked an era in the surgical management of gastric cancer. The concept of radical gastrectomy was not widely accepted in the early twentieth century because operative mortality rates remained high. Further advances in the field of gastric surgery became evident with improvements in anesthesia, postoperative management, and the introduction of antibiotics, which led ultimately to technical modifications and the beginning of modern day gastric oncologic surgery.

Radical gastrectomy: the early American era

At the turn of the twentieth century, the use of radical gastrectomy was limited because of the associated morbidity and mortality. Gastric surgery was most often limited for benign gastric ulcer disease. Balfour presented to the American Surgical Association, on May 2, 1922, a paper titled "Factors Influencing the Life Expectancy of Patients Operated on for Gastric Ulcer" [15]. Through the diligence of his review, Balfour found from information obtained by "case histories, by correspondence, by reexaminations, or by further operation shows very clearly that the most important factor influencing life expectancy...for gastric ulcer is gastric cancer" [15]. Reexamining pathologic biopsy results, Broder showed that 50% of the original tissue specimens from Balfour's study demonstrated malignant histologic changes consistent with gastric cancer. Balfour concluded, "[T]he question of malignant invasion at the operating table makes wide excision of such ulcers of first importance" [15]. The clinical observation that not all gastric ulcers are benign and gross examination is unreliable in the determination of malignancy demonstrated critically the inherent limitations in the treatment of gastric ulcers. In this regard, Balfour proposed wider resection margins to adequately address the possibility that a resected gastric ulcer might be cancerous.

Ranson [16] reported one of the first and largest retrospective studies on the treatment of gastric cancer, which comprised a series from 1934 to 1946 (Table 1). In this study of 1264 patients with gastric cancer, 497 gastric resections were performed, including distal, proximal, and total gastrectomies with few local excisions [16]. In the majority of gastric resections, carcinoma was the most common pathologic diagnosis, with several reported cases of lymphoma and sarcoma. Distal gastrectomy was performed in 80% of gastric resections, with mortality rates as high as 25%. In Ranson's series, the 5-year overall survival was 28% for resectable disease. Autopsy studies demonstrated patterns of local-regional disease recurrence, especially with reference to the increased propensity for perigastric and peripancreatic lymph nodal involvement. Clearly, local-regional recurrence patterns were beginning to be recognized from this early autopsy study.

Table 1
Retrospective historical series: 5-year overall survival rates for gastric cancer resection in the United States (1930s to 1960s)

Study	Date of series	No. of patients in series	No. of gastric resections	Mortality (%)	5-year survival (%)
Ranson [16]	1934–1946	1264	497	25	28
McNeer et al [27]	1931–1950	1623	1315	15	22
Gilbertsen [29]	1936–1963	1983	379	—[a]	10

[a] Overall mortality not reported among the partial and total gastrectomies performed, 18% and 24%, respectively.

The pattern of nodal involvement was not truly appreciated until the work of Coller and colleagues [17]. They studied the regional lymphatic anatomy of the stomach with a technique adopted by Gilchrist and David [18] in their study of rectal lymphatic drainage for rectal cancer. Coller and colleagues examined and mapped out regional lymphatic nodal areas among patients with gastric cancer with reference to tumor location, size, gross morphology, depth of invasion, and histologic tumor differentiation. They reported that 75% of patients had nodal involvement and that gross pathologic findings were unreliable in predicting microscopic disease in the perigastric regional lymph nodes [17]. In addition, resection margins from the duodenum and gastric remnant were positive in 25% of tissue specimens. As also demonstrated by Verbrugghen [19], limited resection was associated with a higher incidence of positive resection margins. Although Coller and colleagues reported margin and nodal status with limited gastric resection, they also provided an anatomic map of the regional lymphatic drainage pathways and corresponding extragastric drainage zones based on the location of the gastric primary cancer. These earlier observations enhanced the understanding of gastric cancer spread, which disseminated mainly through the regional gastric wall lymphatics to regional, perigastric lymph nodes.

The prognosis of gastric cancer in the 1930s and 1940s remained disappointingly poor even among patients with resectable disease [20,21]. Operative mortality rates in many hospitals were reportedly high, with an average risk of 40% in 1940 [22]. McNeer [22] stated, "if the average individual had realized the paucity of his chances for surviving gastrectomy, let alone the disease itself, common sense would have dictated a waiting policy rather than surgical intervention in the treatment of this disease." Although the operative mortality rates were slowly improving, McNeer stated, "there is little reason for smug self-satisfaction among surgeons," and "... that we, as surgeons, must continually subject our technics to critical appraisal" [23]. McNeer and colleagues [23], on the Gastric Service at Memorial Hospital in New York City, performed an autopsy study on patients who had received a partial gastrectomy for cancer. Local-regional failure was detected in 80% of the cases, in which the predominant site of recurrence was identified in the gastric remnant (50%), the perigastric lymph nodes (20.7%), and the duodenal stump (9.8%) [23]. In McNeer's critical reappraisal of the surgical technique, he mentioned that "...surgeons who perform subtotal gastrectomy for duodenal ulcer (disease) apply erroneously the same technic to the treatment of gastric cancer," and cautioned that limited gastric resections were inadequate for suspected malignant disease [23].

Through Pack's earlier work, McNeer proposed wider gastric resection margins with a regional lymphadenectomy in an en bloc fashion and introduced the concept of "extended total gastrectomy" [22,24]. This extirpative resection included a total gastrectomy with resection of the greater and lesser omenta, a splenectomy, distal pancreatectomy, and resection of peritoneum in the lesser sac [25]. This radical change in treatment philosophy was based on his earlier autopsy data, which demonstrated limited local-regional control after subtotal gastrectomy. To further enhance local-regional control, Appleby [26], an associate of McNeer, also incorporated high ligation of the celiac axis in conjunction with an extended total gastrectomy, as a means to facilitate a more complete lymphadenectomy.

McNeer and colleagues [27] reported the end results in the treatment of gastric cancer over a 20-year period (1931–1950). A total of 1623 patients were evaluated for surgical resection. During the first 10 years of the study, 66% of patients underwent an exploratory laparotomy. This rate increased in the later period to 91%. Curative gastric resections were performed in 34% of patients from the entire cohort. During the first 10 years, curative resections were performed only in 16% of patients, but this rate increased to 41.6% in the later period. Among patients who had received a curative resection, subtotal gastrectomy and total gastrectomy were reported in 71% and 29%, respectively. Among the patients from the total gastrectomy group, 49% received the extended total gastrectomy. Of the entire operative series, the postoperative mortality rate was 15% (18% curative versus 13% noncurative). The postoperative mortality rate was 23% for patients who received a total gastrectomy. The 5-year overall survival for all curative resections was 22%. McNeer and coworkers performed a survival analysis on the patients who received a curative resection with regard to primary tumor location, size, Bormann classification, serosal penetration, microscopic grade, and nodal disease. In their analysis, 5-year survival rates were improved for patients who were node-negative, with Bormann type I and II disease, and showed an absence of serosal involvement. Likewise, patients who were node-positive were more likely to have Bormann type III and IV disease with associated serosal involvement. The end result data characterized survival outcomes by demographic variables that provided an insight into the tumor biology for gastric carcinoma.

In the 1950s to 1970s, radical surgical treatment modalities continued to be explored in an effort to improve local-regional control, which previously had appeared compromised by less optimal surgical techniques. The concept of en bloc resection as proposed initially by McNeer offered a surgical solution to disease control, but it was not accepted by practicing gastric surgeons. Although operative mortality rates at this time had not dramatically improved from McNeer's earlier experience, survival rates did gradually improve with the adoption of this more radical concept. In a follow-up study, McNeer and colleagues [28] reported on the outcome of 94 patients who received an elective total gastrectomy, which included resection of contiguous visceral organs (liver, 17, and distal esophagus and colon, 6) from a subset of patients with either proximal or distal gastric cancers. The 5-year survival rates improved from 30% to 43% among patients with distal gastric cancers, but the 5-year survival rates were worse for proximal gastric cancers (19% to 12.7%). The difference observed between patients diagnosed with distal gastric cancer (73%) and those with proximal gastric cancers (43%) was a higher rate of nodal disease. Nodal positivity was dependent on the extent of lymphadenectomy, such that 25% of patients who received a partial gastrectomy and limited lymphadenectomy were more likely to be node-negative, as opposed to patients who received an extended total gastrectomy, in which nodal disease was more commonly identified. The survival benefit was attributed to the more extended procedure in that patients with limited resection would invariably have disease left behind. Thus, the radical surgical approach at that time favored an extended total gastrectomy for least distal gastric cancers but was considered ineffective for proximal gastric cancers.

Although the concept of radical gastrectomy seemed promising for a subset of patients, results were difficult to reproduce, and trepidation was still evident in these earlier series. Gilbertsen [29] examined the concept of radical resections in a large retrospective analysis that compared mortality rates and 5-year survival rates among 1983 patients at the University of Minnesota, from 1936 to 1963. Longmire [30], in an article titled "Gastric Carcinoma: Is Radical Gastrectomy Worthwhile?" reviewed this question and concluded that total gastrectomy should only be performed under specific indications and that subtotal gastrectomy instead of total gastrectomy should be performed for antral gastric cancers. Gilbersten failed to show a survival advantage with the 5-year overall survival rate of 10.2%. The operative mortality rates increased with radical surgery from 22.5% to 33.3% among patients who had received both a total gastrectomy and lymphadenectomy. Likewise, the mortality rates also increased from 13.3% to 25.6% when lymphadenectomy was performed with a partial gastrectomy. Despite wider resection margins and extended lymphadenectomy, patients with lymph node-positive disease in Gilbertsen's series did not benefit as well as McNeer's later experience. However, Gilbertsen concluded that, "…patient survival [is] not likely to occur as a result of fabrication of larger operations and more extensive lymph node dissections to replace existing procedures for routine use in the treatment of stomach cancer patients." [29].

Subtotal versus total gastrectomy: a more contemporary prospective

Historical surgical series were nonrandomized, retrospective reviews of the benefits of total gastrectomy. Shiu and colleagues [31] performed a retrospective analysis at Memorial Sloan Kettering Cancer Center (MSKCC) on survival outcome based on the extent of gastric resection for gastric carcinoma. They reported their experience over a 20-year period (1960–1980) with 210 patients who had received a curative gastric resection. Patients in the total gastrectomy group showed a median survival that was not improved compared with the subtotal gastrectomy group with a median survival at 16.9 versus 60.3 months, respectively [31]. This significantly decreased survival rate was found among patients who had larger lesions, those with a more proximal tumor, and those who had received a splenectomy and distal pancreatectomy. A multivariate analysis showed that the location (proximal versus distal), extent of nodal disease (≥ 3 lymph nodes), positive resection margins, extent of lymphadenectomy, and gastrectomy were all independently negative prognostic variables. Although the study was unable to confirm a survival benefit, a higher proportion of patients who had received a total gastrectomy had proximal gastric cancers with more advanced staged disease that often required en bloc visceral organ resection to achieve a curative resection.

The first prospective trial, performed in Hong Kong, compared a subtotal gastrectomy arm with a total gastrectomy arm for distal gastric cancers. Robertson and colleagues [32] randomized 55 patients into a subtotal gastrectomy (25 patients) arm and a total gastrectomy (30 patients) arm. The patients in the subtotal gastrectomy arm had a 6-cm wide proximal gastric resection margin with resection of N1 perigastric lymph nodes. Patients in the total gastrectomy arm had resections of the greater and lesser omenta, spleen, distal pancreas, and N2 lymph nodes. Median survival was not improved for the patients in the total gastrectomy arm (922 days for R3 versus 1511 days for R1, $P = 0.04$). Instead, patients who were randomized to the subtotal gastrectomy arm achieved a survival benefit without the greater need for blood transfusion requirements and associated morbidities.

Two prospective European trials have compared subtotal gastrectomy and total gastrectomy for distal gastric tumors. In the French trial, Gouzi and colleagues [33] randomized 169 patients and found no difference in 5-year survival rates. However, the trial was criticized for lack of statistical power and faulty analysis. In the larger, multicenter Italian trial by Bozzetti and colleagues [34], 622 patients were randomized into two treatments arms: subtotal gastrectomy (319 patients) and total gastrectomy (303 patients). In this trial, both gastrectomy arms received a comparable D2 lymphadenectomy. The 5-year overall survival was 64%, and no survival advantage was conferred in the total gastrectomy arm by multivariate analysis. Prognostic variables that were independently associated with an increased risk of death included the level of invasion, need for en bloc organ resection (spleen or additional organ), and the ratio of metastatic lymph nodes to negative nodes ($\geq 25\%$). Interestingly, positive resection margins were not independently associated with worse outcome, which also was reported by Kim and colleagues [35] in patients who had greater than 5 positive lymph nodes. This well-designed Italian trial revealed comparable survival results between both treatment arms that favored a subtotal gastrectomy for distal gastric cancers. Also, Bozzetti and colleagues demonstrated that extended lymphadenectomy was not compromised by a subtotal gastrectomy.

Unlike distal gastric cancers, the optimal surgical treatment for proximal gastric cancers remained a challenge. The type of gastrectomy and extent of gastric margins remains controversial. In a retrospective study, Papachristou and Fortner [36] found that survival for early staged disease (stages I and II) depended on the extent of resection in favor of an extended total gastrectomy; however, in advanced staged disease (stages III and IV), the extent of resection had no influence on survival, despite a higher local recurrence rate that occurred in early staged disease treated with a more conservative proximal gastrectomy. In another series from MSKCC, Harrison and colleagues [37] reevaluated the issue for optimal resection margins in proximal gastric cancers. From their prospective database, they identified 391 patients with proximal gastric cancers, who underwent resections between 1985 and 1995. They excluded 293 patients who had undergone an esophagogastrectomy and analyzed 98 cases that had received either a proximal gastrectomy (65) or a total gastrectomy (33). The 5-year overall survival was 43% and 41%, respectively, without a significant difference. Local recurrence and time to local recurrence were not significantly different. Patients who had received a total gastrectomy were more likely to have had higher staged disease. Unlike the distal cohort, the extent of surgical resection margins for proximal gastric cancers has not been confirmed in a prospective randomized fashion.

Radical lymphadenectomy

Lymphadenectomy for gastric carcinoma: trends and rationale

Today, few centers in the United States and Western countries regularly incorporate extended lymphadenectomy in their standard surgical practices for curative gastric resections. Wanebo and colleagues [38] have reported in a retrospective study that the extent of lymph node dissection was mainly limited to the perigastric lymph nodes, in which only 4.7% of patients with R0 resections had received a more extended lymph node dissection. MacDonald and colleagues [39], in the Intergroup trial, reported similar lymphadenectomy rates with just 10% of patients receiving a D2 lymphadenectomy and 54% receiving a D0 dissection. Although relapse-free survival rates (19 months in the surgery group versus 30 months in the adjuvant chemo-radiation therapy group, $P < 0.001$) and overall survival rates (27 months in the surgery group versus 36 months in the adjuvant chemo-radiation therapy group, $P = 0.005$) were improved by adjuvant chemo-radiation therapy, the trial failed to incorporate surgical quality control measures to standardized the surgical treatment. This is in direct contrast to the prototypical adjuvant or neoadjuvant surgical trial, as exemplified in the Dutch Rectal Cancer Study, in which optimally resected rectal cancer by total mesorectal excision was combined with preoperative radiation. Compared with the Intergroup trial, Kapiteijn and colleagues [40] demonstrated benefits with neoadjuvant radiation in optimally resected rectal cancer, in contrast to the Intergroup trial, in which more than half of the patients received a less than optimal surgical resection. Although fewer US and Western centers regularly perform extended lymph node dissections for gastric cancer, the standard of care as established by the Intergroup trial brings into question the benefits of adding either a neoadjuvant or adjuvant treatment protocol in optimally resected gastric cancer patients.

In contrast, Japanese centers and few specialized Western centers have demonstrated comparable morbidity and mortality rates between both a D1 and D2 dissection [8]. However, few Western centers have been able to reproduce these results, in contrast to the Japanese and German series, with current US adjuvant data supporting a more limited lymphadenectomy [38,39,41–43]. Two recent prospective trials have failed to demonstrate a survival benefit because of the higher morbidity and mortality rates observed among patients who received a D2 dissection with combined splenectomy or distal pancreatectomy [44,45]. In addition, Dent and colleagues [46] have reported that patients with a higher body mass index had higher morbidity and mortality rates. However, this association was not a factor that adversely affected outcome between two Japanese centers in Yokohama and MSKCC; instead, the differences reported were explained mainly by tumor location and stage [8]. In the current Western series, the predominant demographic variables that have contributed to the observed differences have been related to a higher incidence of proximal gastric cancers, more advanced disease at diagnosis (stage III and IV), and differences among Japanese and American pathologists with regard to the diagnostic criteria used to diagnose carcinoma [4,8,38,47].

The major rationale for using extended lymphadenectomy for gastric cancer has been the historical lack of local-regional control with more limited surgery. Recurrence patterns were predominantly local-regional, but a more current series has demonstrated distal failure as the first site of disease recurrence [48,49]. The major impetus for extended lymph node dissection has been the eradication of occult regional nodal disease, thus minimizing and abrogating the development of local-regional recurrence. This surgical treatment philosophy is based on the classic Halstedian model of tumor metastases [50]. Based on this model, lymph nodes function as mere Millipore-type filters, trapping neoplastic cells before systemic dissemination. The eradication of regional nodal basins with radical lymphadenectomy has been proposed to eliminate regional disease and improve local-regional control. Currently, lymph node status functions merely as prognostic indicators, which represent the "speedometer of the oncologic engine" [50,51].

The National Surgical Adjuvant Breast Project B4 trial [52] confirmed this notion and demonstrated equivalent survival rates among women randomized between a modified radical mastectomy, a simple mastectomy with adjuvant axillary radiotherapy, and simple mastectomy. A recent 20-year follow-up still demonstrated that overall survival had not been adversely influenced by axillary treatment, which indicated that nodal status was a mere indicator but not the governor of overall survival. This result also was observed in patients who received surgical treatment for gastric, colorectal, breast, or lung carcinoma who had more than five positive lymph nodes, underwent radical treatment, and received no affect on overall survival, with less than a 2% 5-year survival rate [50,53]. As a consequence, there has been major paradigm shift in the philosophy of breast cancer treatment with the introduction of lymphatic mapping and sentinel lymph node biopsy. Although obligatory radical lymphadenectomies were a necessary component in the surgical management of breast cancer in the era of radical breast surgery, this procedure has now been supplanted by selective lymphadenectomy in breast cancer patients; the reliability of this technique for gastric cancer remains to be determined, and the extent of lymphadenectomy continues to be debated.

Lymphadenectomy in gastric cancer: Japanese guidelines

The Japanese began to adopt radical resections in their surgical armamentarium in gastric surgery in the 1960s. The guidelines that were established by the Japanese Research Society for Gastric Cancer (JRSGC) issued "the General Rules for Gastric Cancer Study in Surgery and Pathology" [54], which was published initially in Japan in 1962 and subsequently translated into an English version and adopted by Western surgeons. The Japanese identified lymphatic nodal regions through dye injection studies and classified draining lymphatic basins into 16 stations (Fig. 2). The JRSGC established surgical quality control measures that allowed Japanese surgeons to monitor the quality of resections and standardized the pathologic nomenclature. Nagata and colleagues [55] found that, as Japanese surgeons accepted and adopted the established rules, resection of N1 and N2 nodal groups increased from 1.1% in the early 1960s to 87% in the 1970s, at Kyushu University. During this same time period, curative gastric resection rates also increased from 28% to 85%. This dramatic increase in curative resection rates also was accompanied by their implementation of a national screening program, which resulted in an increase in the proportion of early gastric cancers diagnosed, with a significant reduction in the incidence of advanced gastric cancers (stages III and IV) [56]. The guidelines established by the JRSGC and the national screening program prompted many Japanese surgeons to accept D2 lymphadenectomy as the standard of care.

Lymphadenectomy in gastric cancer: Japanese retrospective series

In the last several decades, the Japanese have demonstrated improvements in outcome for gastric cancer treatments with D2 lymphadenectomy. Their experience has been based largely on retrospective studies. An earlier Japanese retrospective study documented a 5-year survival benefit for D2 lymphadenectomy compared with historical controls, that is, patients who

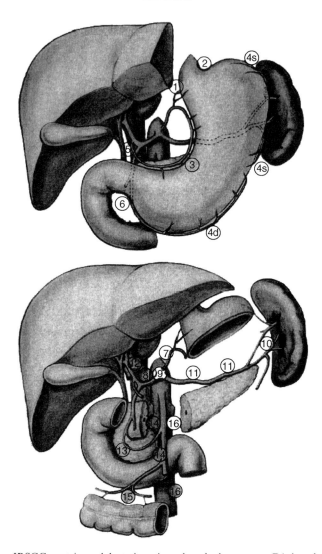

Fig. 2. The JRSGC gastric nodal stations in a lymphadenectomy. D1 lymphadenectomy removal of stations 1 to 6. D2 lymphadenectomy removal of stations 1 to 6 and 7 to 12. D3 lymphadenectomy removal of 1 to 12 plus para-aortic lymph nodes. (*From* Hartgrink HH, van de Velde CJH, Putter H, et al. Extended lymph node dissection for gastric cancer: who may benefit? final results of the randomized Dutch Gastric Cancer Group Trial. J Clin Ortho 2004;22(11):1–9; with permission.)

had traditionally received a D1 lymphadenectomy [57]. Kodama and colleagues [57] have reported a 5-year survival benefit for D2 lymphadenectomy in patients with positive nodal disease or serosal involvement. Other large Japanese series have shown impressive 5-year survival rates, stage for stage, compared with American series (Table 2) [41,42].

Table 2
Comparision of 5-year survival rates for gastric resection between Western and Eastern countries by stage

	No. of patient in series	Stages (%)					
		IA	IB	II	IIIA	IIIB	IV
United States							
Wanebo, et al [38][a]	10,237	50	—	29	13	—	3
Hundahl	32,532	78	58	34	20	8	7
Germany							
Siewert, et al [62] ≤25 LN	404	81	69	29	24	20	22
≥25 LN	778	84	68	57*	32**	14	13
Japan							
Maruyama [41][a]	12,535	96	—	70	36	—	23
Ichikawa, et al [42] >15 LN	587	95	86	71	59	35	17

Abbreviation: LN, lymph nodes.
[a] Staging grouped by stage I, II, III, and IV.
* $P < 0.001$; ** $P = 0.035$.
Data from Hundahl SA, Phillips JL, Menck HR. The National Cancer Database report on the poor survival of US gastric carcinoma patients treated with gastrectomy. Cancer 2000;88: 921–34.

Since the JRSGC was established, Japanese centers have routinely performed D2 rather than D1 lymphadenectomies for curative gastric resections. Japanese investigators have not conducted prospective trials that compare the survival benefits between D1 and D2 lymphadenectomy. Because of their success with D2 lymphadenectomy, they have examined the role of a more extended lymphadenectomy, D3 dissection. However, three retrospective series failed to demonstrate a 5-year overall survival benefit when D3 lymphadenectomy was compared with a D2 lymphadenectomy [58–60]. Currently, the Japanese Clinical Oncology Group [61] has conducted a preliminary prospective trial that has evaluated the feasibility and safety for a D3 lymphadenectomy. These preliminary data have shown comparable morbidity and mortality rates, but long-term outcome data are forthcoming.

Lymphadenectomy in gastric cancer: a German nonrandomized series

One of the first prospective, nonrandomized trials that became available has compared D1 with D2 lymphadenectomy. Siewart and colleagues [62] organized a large multiple center trial modeled after the JRSGC rules that incorporated en bloc D2 lymphadenectomy in the management of gastric carcinoma. A total of 1654 patients were included in the study, in which 1182 of the 1654 patients (71.5%) received an R0 resection. The study design addressed surgical and pathologic quality control measures that standardized the extent and quality of lymphadenectomy and standardized the gross and histopathologic assessment of the resected tissue specimens. D2 lymphadenectomy was defined by the average number of lymph nodes expected in the upper abdominal compartments, with greater than 25 lymph nodes for a D2 dissection and less than 25 lymph nodes for a D1 dissection. However, the level or extent of lymphadenectomy was left to the discretion of the operating surgeon. Approximately 66% of patients received a D2 lymphadenectomy. Mortality rates between D1 and D2 resections were not significantly different (5.2% for D1 versus 5.0% for D2). Patients with stage II (pT2, N1 and pT3, and N0) disease showed improved 10-year overall survival rates with extended lymphadenectomy (19.9% for D1 versus 49.2% for D2; $P \leq 0.001$), whereas patients with stage IIIA disease initially achieved an improved 5-year overall survival benefit, but survival failed to remain significant at 10 years. Multivariate analysis showed that the extent of lymph node dissection proved to be an independent prognostic indicator. Although Siewart's [62] study was not a randomized trial, it at least showed a survival benefit for a selected subset of patients with stage II disease in an otherwise well-conducted surgical study.

Lymphadenectomy in gastric cancer: prospective randomize series

In a report from South Africa, Dent and colleagues [46] reported the first randomized prospective trial that compared D1 and D2 lymphadenectomy. The authors evaluated 603 patients with gastric cancer, of whom 403 patients proceeded to undergo laparotomy and 43 patients underwent curative gastric resection. Patients were excluded from the study if they had evidence of peritoneal involvement, distant metastasis, or direct tumor invasion (T4 lesions). Patients who fulfilled the eligibility criteria (T1–3, N0–2, and M0) were randomized at surgery to two treatment arms (22 patients in the D1 group versus 21 patients in the D2 group). The accrual was very limited, and the study lacked statistical power; 3-year survival rates were unaffected by the level of lymphadenectomy (78% for D1 versus 76% for D2; $P \leq 0.77$). Dent and colleagues reported no hospital deaths, but patients randomized to the D2 arm required a higher number of transfusions, longer operative times, and longer hospital stay. Clearly, the South African study failed to show a survival advantage in favor of an extended lymphadenectomy, but it showed that hospital mortality was not higher in the D2 arm. The authors concluded that D2 lymphadenectomy should be performed only in a clinical trial setting.

Since the South African trial, survival benefits associated with extended lymph node dissection have been confirmed only by retrospective data. The South African trial was underpowered and lacking in design. In the United Kingdom, the Medical Research Council (MRC)-gastric cancer Surgical Trial (STO1) and the Dutch Gastric Cancer Group each designed two randomized prospective trials that evaluated survival benefits for a D2 lymphadenectomy [63,64]. Both of these trials were modeled after the JRSGC guidelines, which included as a standard component of their D2 lymphadenectomy resection of the distal pancreas and spleen to facilitate dissection of the lymph node groups along the designated N2 stations.

Cuschieri and colleagues [64] reported the MRC-STO1 results in 1996, with a follow-up report in 1999. The morbidity (28% for D1 versus 46% for D2; $P \leq 0.001$) and mortality (6.5% for D1 versus 13% for D2; $P = 0.04$) rates were significantly higher in the D2 arm compared with the D1 arm [44,64]. The 5-year overall survival rates in the D1 (35%) and D2 (33%) arms were not significantly different ($P = 0.43$) (Fig. 3). Likewise, Cuschieri and colleagues reported no significant difference ($P = 0.79$) between the recurrence-free survival rates. Surgeons in this study had received video-taped instructions on the extent and performance of the lymph node dissection. Despite the quality assurance, noncompliance and contamina-tion were reported among the patients in both treatment arms. In the D1 arm, 27% of patients underwent a splenectomy and 4% received pan-creaticosplenectomy compared with the D2 arm, in which a combined panreaticosplenectomy was performed in 57% of the resections. In addition, some patients assigned to the D1 arm had N2 lymph nodes sampled, whereas some of the patients in the D2 arm had N3 nodes sampled [64]. Among 375 patients reported in the study, 310 patients had less than 26 harvested lymph nodes (165 patients for D1 versus 145 for D2) compared with only 65 patients in whom more than 26 lymph nodes were resected (19 patients for D1 versus 46 patients for D2). In their multivariate analysis, splenectomy or distal pancreatectomy were independently associated with

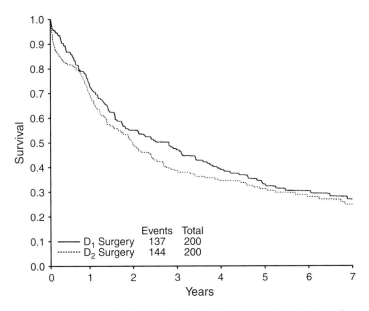

Fig. 3. Comparison of UK Medical Research Council 5-year overall survival rates between D1 (35%) and D2 (33%) lymphadenectomy ($P = 0.43$). (*Data from* Cuschieri A, Weeden S, Fielding J, et al. Patient survival after D1 and D2 resections for gastric cancer: long-term results of the MRC randomised surgical trial. Br J Cancer 1999;79(9/10):1522–30.)

an increased hazard ratio. In conclusion, the data favored a more limited surgical approach with significantly less morbidity and mortality when pancreaticosplenectomy was not included in the lymphadenectomy. The authors acknowledged that patients may have achieved a survival benefit without pancreaticosplenectomy. However future prospective trials will be needed too adequately address this hypothesis.

In the Netherlands, the Dutch Gastric Cancer Group recently reported long-term overall survival, relapse-free survival and morbidity and mortality rates for extended lymphadenectomy in their multicenter trial [45]. The Dutch trial as well as the MRC trial used the JRSGC guidelines and rules in their design. Surgical quality control measures included surgeons receiving instructions from both a videotape and the presence of an expert Japanese surgeon in the operating room. Supervision was closely monitored during the initial 4-month training period and then regularly thereafter. One of eight regional surgeons who had been trained by an expert Japanese surgeon regularly attended D2 dissections. The morbidity (25% for D1 versus 43% for D2; $P \leq 0.001$) and mortality (4% for D1 versus 10% for D2; $P = 0.004$) rates were significantly higher for the D2 lymphadenectomy arm when associated with splenectomy (37%) or distal pancreatectomy (30%) [45]. Overall survival differences were small and not significantly different at 5 years' (45% for D1 versus 47% for D2) and at 11 years' follow-up (31% for D1 versus 35% for D2; $P = 0.53$) (Fig. 4) [45,63]. Although a subgroup analysis showed a trend toward improved survival among patients with N2 disease, an 11-year survival rate of 21% was observed in the D2 arm, but compared with the D1 arm there were no long-term survivors [45]. The

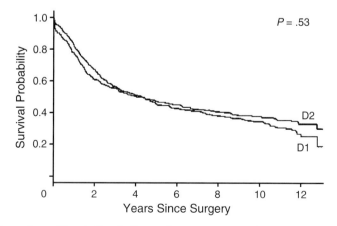

Fig. 4. Comparison of Dutch Gastric Cancer Group 11-year overall survival rates between D1 (30%) and D2 (35%) lymphadenectomy ($P = 0.53$). (*Data from* Hartgrink HH, van de Velde CJH, Putter H, et al. Extended lymph node dissection for gastric cancer: who may benefit? final results of the randomized Dutch Gastric Cancer Group Trial. J Clin Ortho 2004;22(11):1–9.)

Dutch Gastric Study Group concluded that long-term survival was not improved with extended lymph node dissection.

Like the MRC trial, the Dutch trial also reported issues with contamination and noncompliance violations, which were reported less frequently than in the MRC trial; 11% of D1 patients had a splenectomy, and 3% of D1 patients had a distal pancreatectomy [44,45]. The Dutch trial favored a more limited D1 dissection, because the associated morbidity and mortality rates probably obviated any survival benefit that might have been achieved if pancreaticosplenectomy were not performed in conjunction with the standard D2 dissection. Like the MRC trial, the Dutch designed surgical quality control measures into the trial to standardize and ensure the adequacy lymphadenectomy in the D2 arm. Despite their efforts, protocol violations, which were less frequently reported, made direct comparisons difficult to interpret because of the extent of contamination that was recognized in both trials. Future investigators will need to be very cognizant of this issue to avoid cross-contamination and to perform standard D2 lymphadenectomy trials without pancreaticosplenectomy. Although a purely surgical trial may never be performed, the validity of D2 lymphadenectomy will continue to be debated, especially with the advent of increasing reliance of adjuvant or neoadjuvant regimens to compensate for less radical gastric surgery, as demonstrated by the Intergroup investigator (Fig. 5).

Although the British and Dutch investigators were unable to demonstrate a survival advantage in favor of a D2 lymphadenectomy, Japanese and German authors' data continue to support extended lymph node dissection [41,42,62]. A major criticism of the MRC and Dutch trials has been the increased morbidity and mortality rates associated with pancreaticosple-

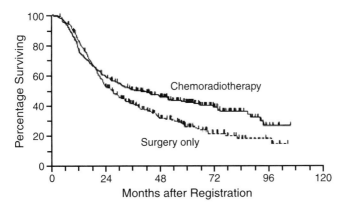

Fig. 5. Comparison of Intergroup 3-year overall survival rates between adjuvant chemo-radiation (Chemoradiotherapy) arm (50%) and surgery (Surgery only) arm (41%) ($P = 0.005$). (*Data from* MacDonald JS, Smalley SR, Benedetti J, et al. Chemoradiotherapy after surgery compared with surgery alone for adenocarcinoma of the stomach or gastroesophageal junction. N Engl J Med 2001;345(10):725–30.)

nectomy. This has prompted critical reappraisal of the need to perform a splenectomy or distal pancreatectomy as part of the D2 lymphadenectomy. Because recent retrospective data have not demonstrated a survival benefit in the routine performance of pancreaticosplenectomy, as required originally by the JRSGC in their description of D2 dissections, Japanese centers have been prompted to avoid pancreaticosplenectomy as part of their D2 lymphadenectomy [65–67]. Despite a 10% incidence of splenic nodal involvement, Csendes and colleagues [68] were unable to document a survival advantage (36% for spleen-preserving 5-year overall survival (OS) versus 42% for splenectomy 5-year OS; $P \geq 0.5$) that favored splenectomy. In addition, the number of lymph nodes removed and the ratio of metastatic lymph nodes to normal lymph nodes have appeared as better prognostic indicators than the more traditional concept of nodal involvement based on lymph node station [46,62,69–72]. As a result, changes in the American Joint Committee on Cancer have modified the TNM staging system that now requires removal of greater than 15 lymph nodes for adequate staging, because the extent of nodal involvement is an independent prognostic indicator [73].

Lymphadenectomy in gastric cancer: early gastric cancer

Current prospective data has not supported D2 lymphadenectomy, and the adverse affects associated with pancreaticosplenectomy have redefined surgical treatment options for gastric cancer. This data has become more apparent with the surgical treatment for early gastric cancers (EGC), which the Japanese have described as a disease limited to the mucosa or submucosa, independent of nodal disease [56]. Survival rates for ECG have been favorable with greater than 90% 5-year survival rates [41,42]. Currently, Japanese surgeons are performing more conservative resections for ECG [74,75]. In a Western series, Hochwald and colleagues [76] have examined clinicopathologic features that are used to predict nodal involvement. In their prospective database, 165 patients were identified with pT1 disease. Overall survival was 88% (91% survival in node-negative patients versus 78% survival in node-positive patients). On multivariate analysis, prognostic factors that were predictive of nodal disease included submucosal invasion, vascular invasion, and primary tumor size. Patients who had no submucosal invasion and a primary tumor size less than 4.5 cm had a nodal positivity rate of 4%. The authors speculated that for a subset of patients with ECG, a more conservative resection without lymphadenectomy may be considered [76].

Summary

The history of gastric cancer surgery has taught us many lessons. The trend toward a more radical philosophy in the surgical treatment of gastric cancer emerged mainly around World War II in the United States. The limitation imposed by radical resections was attributed mostly to increased postoperative morbidity and mortality rates with marginal survival outcomes. The implementation of standardized surgical quality control measures by the Japanese created a standard surgical approach with defined nodal stations and a common nomenclature. The limitations imposed by retrospective data and the failure of two recent prospective trials have influenced Western surgeons' reluctance to pursue further investigation in the surgical merits of D2 lymphadenectomy in the presence of improved adjuvant chemo-radiation therapy regimens and now enhanced interest in the development of neoadjuvant protocols. These factors have changed the attitude of practicing surgeons to adopt a more cautionary and conservative approach in oncologic management of gastric cancer.

References

[1] Mayer RJ, Rosoff CB, Feldman MI. Cancers of the stomach. In: Cancer: a manual for practitioners. 5th edition. Boston: American Cancer Society; 1978. p. 159.
[2] Jemal A, Murray T, Samuels A, et al. Cancer statistic 2003. CA Cancer J Clin 2003;53:5–26.
[3] Blot WJ, Devesa SS, Kneller RW, et al. Rising incidence of adenocarcinoma of the esophagus and gastric cardia. JAMA 1991;265(10):1287–9.
[4] Devesa SS, Blot WJ, Fraumeni JF. Changing patterns in the incidence of esophageal and gastric carcinoma in the United States. Cancer 1998;83(10):2049–53.
[5] Locke GR, Talley NJ, Carpenter HA, et al. Changes in the site- and histology-specific incidence of gastric cancer during a 50-year period. Gastroenterology 1995;109:1750–6.
[6] Meyers WC, Damiano RJ, Postlethwait RW, et al. Adenocarcinoma of the stomach: changing patterns over the last 4 decades. Ann Surg 1987;205(1):1–8.
[7] Bollschweiler E, Boettcher K, Hoelscher AH, et al. Is the prognosis for Japanese and German patients with gastric cancer really different. Cancer 1993;71(10):2918–25.
[8] Noguchi Y, Yoshikawa T, Tsuburaya A, et al. Is gastric carcinoma different between Japan and the United States. Cancer 2000;89(11):2237–46.
[9] Wanebo HJ, Turk PS. General surgical principles in gastrointestinal cancer. In: Wanebo HJ, editor. Surgery for gastrointestinal cancer. New York: Lippincott-Raven; 1997. p. 19.
[10] Lawrence W. Gastric cancer. In: McKenna RJ, Murphy GP, editors. Fundamentals of surgical oncology. New York: Macmillan; 1986. p. 657.
[11] Siewert RJ, Hoelscher AH, Billroth I. Gastrectomy. In: Nyhus LM, Baker RJ, editors. Master of surgery. 2nd edition. Boston: Little, Brown and Company; 1992. p. 639.
[12] Hoerr SO, Steiger E, Billroth I. Gastrectomy. In: Nyhus LM, Baker RJ, editors. Master of surgery. 2nd edition. Boston: Little, Brown and Company; 1992. p. 649.
[13] Shackelford RT, Dugan HJ. The stomach and duodenum. In: Shackelford RT, editor. Surgery of the alimentary tract, volume 1. Philadelphia: WB Saunders Co; 1965. p. 375.
[14] Jewkes A, Taylor EW, Fielding JWL, et al. Radical total gastrectomy for carcinoma. In: Nyhus LM, Baker RJ, editors. Master of surgery. 2nd edition. Boston: Little, Brown and Company; 1992. p. 721.
[15] Balfour DC. Factors influencing the life expectancy of patients operated on for gastric ulcer. Ann Surg 1922;77:405–8.
[16] Ranson HK. Cancer of the stomach. J Am Coll Surg (Surg Gynecol Obstet) 1953;96:275–87.
[17] Coller FA, Kay EB, McIntyre RS. Regional lymphatic metastases of carcinoma of the stomach. Arch Surg 1942;43:748–61.

[18] Gilchrist RK, David VC. Lymphatic spread of carcinoma of the rectum. Ann Surg 1938;108: 621–42.

[19] Verbrugghen A. Intramural extension of gastric carcinoma. Arch Surg 1934;28:566.

[20] Lahey FH. Complete removal of the stomach for malignancy with report of five surgically successful cases. J Am Coll Surg (Surg Gynecol Obstet) 1938;67:213–23.

[21] Graham RR. Total gastrectomy for carcinoma of the stomach. Arch Surg 1943;46:907–17.

[22] McNeer G, Sunderland DA, McInnes G, et al. A more thorough operation for gastric cancer: anatomical basis and description of technique. Cancer 1951;4:957–67.

[23] McNeer G, VandenBerg H, Donn FY, et al. A critical evaluation of subtotal gastrectomy for cure of cancer of the stomach. Ann Surg 1951;134:2–7.

[24] Pack GT, McNeer G, Booher RJ. Principles governing total gastrectomy. Arch Surg 1947; 24:457–85.

[25] McNeer G, Lawrence W, Ortega LG, et al. Early results of extended total gastrectomy for cancer. Cancer 1956;9:1153–9.

[26] Appleby LH. The coeliac axis in the expansion of the operation for gastric carcinoma. Cancer 1953;6(4):704–7.

[27] McNeer G, Lawrence W, Ashley MP, et al. End results in the treatment of gastric cancer. Surgery 1958;43(6):879–96.

[28] McNeer G, Bowden L, Booher RJ, et al. Elective total gastrectomy for cancer of the stomach: end results. Ann Surg 1974;180(2):252–6.

[29] Gilbertsen VA. Results of treatment of stomach cancer: an appraisal of efforts for more extensive surgery and a report of 1,983 cases. Cancer 1969;23(6):1305–8.

[30] Longmire WP. Gastric carcinoma: is radical gastrectomy worthwhile? Ann R Coll Surg Engl 1980;62:25–30.

[31] Shiu MH, Moore E, Sanders M, et al. Influence of the extent of resection on survival after curative treatment of gastric carcinoma: a retrospective multivariate analysis. Arch Surg 1987;122:1347–51.

[32] Robertson CS, Chung SCS, Woods SDS, et al. A prospective randomized trial comparing R1 subtotal gastrectomy with R3 total gastrectomy for antral cancer. Ann Surg 1994;220(2): 176–82.

[33] Gouzi JL, Huguier M, Fagniez PL, et al. Total versus subtotal gastrectomy for adenocarcinoma of the gastric antrum. Ann Surg 1989;209:162–6.

[34] Bozzetti F, Marubini E, Bonfanti G, et al. Subtotal versus total gastrectomy for gastric cancer. Ann Surg 1999;230(2):170–8.

[35] Kim SH, Karpeh MS, Klimstra DS, et al. Effect of microscopic resection line disease on gastric cancer survival. J Gastrointest Surg 1999;3(1):24–33.

[36] Papachristou DN, Fortner JG. Adenocarcinoma of the gastric cardia: the choice of gastrectomy. Ann Surg 1980;192(1):58–64.

[37] Harrison LE, Karpeh MS, Brennan MB. Total gastrectomy is not necessary for proximal gastric cancer. Surgery 1998;123(2):127–30.

[38] Wanebo HJ, Kennedy BJ, Chmiel J, et al. Cancer of the stomach: a patient care study by the American College of Surgeons. Ann Surg 1993;218(5):583–92.

[39] MacDonald JS, Smalley SR, Benedetti J, et al. Chemoradiotherapy after surgery compared with surgery alone for adenocarcinoma of the stomach or gastroesophageal junction. N Engl J Med 2001;345(10):725–30.

[40] Kapiteijn E, Marujnen CAM, Nagtegaal ID, et al. Preoperative radiotherapy combined with total mesorectal excision for respectable rectal cancer. N Engl J Med 2001;345(9):638–45.

[41] Maruyama K, Okabayashi K, Kinoshita T. Progress in gastric cancer surgery in Japan and its limits of radicality. World J Surg 1987;11:418–25.

[42] Ichikura T, Tominmatsu S, Uefuji K, et al. Evaluation of the new American Joint Committee on Cancer/International Union Against Cancer classification of lymph node metastasis from gastric carcinoma in comparison with the Japanese classification. Cancer 1999;86:553–8.

[43] Roder JD, Bottcher K, Busch R, et al. Classification of regional lymph node metastasis from gastric carcinoma. Cancer 1998;82:621–31.

[44] Cuschieri A, Weeden S, Fielding J, et al. Patient survival after D1 and D2 resections for gastric cancer: long-term results of the MRC randomized surgical trial. Br J Cancer 1999; 79(9/10):1522–30.

[45] Hartgrink HH, van de Velde CJH, Putter H, et al. Extended lymph node dissection for gastric cancer: who may benefit? final results of the randomized Dutch Gastric Cancer Group Trial. J Clin Orthod 2004;22(11):1–9.

[46] Dent DM, Madden MV, Price SK. Randomized comparison of R1 and R2 gastrectomy for gastric carcinoma. Br J Surg 1988;75:110–2.

[47] Schlemper RJ, Itabashi M, Kato Y, et al. Differences in diagnostic criteria for gastric carcinoma between Japanese and Western pathologists. Lancet 1997;349:1725–9.

[48] MacDonald JS, Steele G, Gunderson LL. Carcinoma of the stomach. In: DeVita V, Hellman S, Rosenberg SA, editors. Principles and practices of oncology. 2nd edition. Philadelphia: JB Lippincott; 1989. p. 675.

[49] D'Angelica M, Gonen M, Brennan MF, et al. Patterns of initial recurrence in completely resected gastric adenocarcinoma. Ann Surg 2004;240(5):808–16.

[50] Cady B. Basic principles in surgical oncology. Arch Surg 1997;132:338–46.

[51] Cady B. Fundamentals of contemporary surgical oncology: biologic principles and the threshold concept govern treatment and outcomes. J Am Coll Surg 2001;192(6):777–92.

[52] Fisher B, Jeong JH, Anderson S, et al. Twenty-five year follow-up of a randomized trial comparing radical mastectomy, total mastectomy and total mastectomy followed by irradiation. N Engl J Med 2002;347(8):567–76.

[53] Harvey HD, Auchincloss H. Metastases to lymph nodes from carcinomas that were arrested. Cancer 1968;21:684–91.

[54] Japanese Research Society for Gastric Cancer. The general rules for the gastric cancer study in surgery and pathology. Jpn J Surg 1981;11(2):127–39.

[55] Nagata T, Ikeda M, Nakayama F. Changing state of gastric cancer in Japan. Am J Surg 1983;145:226–33.

[56] Murakami T. Early cancer of the stomach. World J Surg 1979;3:685.

[57] Kodama Y, Sugimachi K, Soejima K, et al. Evaluation of extensive lymph node dissection for carcinoma of the stomach. World J Surg 1981;5:241–8.

[58] Mine M, Majima S, Harada M, et al. End results of gastrectomy for gastric cancer: Effect of extensive lymph node dissection. Surgery 1970;68:753–8.

[59] Majima S, Etani S, Fujita Y, et al. Evaluation of extended lymph node dissection for gastric cancer. Jpn J Surg 1972;2:1–6.

[60] Kaibura N, Sumi K, Yonekawa M, et al. Does extensive dissection of lymph nodes improve the results of surgical treatment of gastric cancer. Am J Surg 1990;159:218–21.

[61] Sano T, Sasako M, Yamamoto S, Nashimoto A, et al. Gastric cancer surgery: morbidity and mortality results from a prospective randomized controlled trial comparing D2 and extended para-aotic lymphadenectomy: Japan Clinical Oncology Group Study 9501. J Clin Oncol 2004;22(4):2767–73.

[62] Siewert JR, Bottcher K, Stein HJ, et al. Relevant prognostic factors in gastric cancer: ten-year results of the German Gastric Cancer Study. Ann Surg 1998;228(4):449–61.

[63] Bonenkamp JJ, Sasako M, van de Velde CJH. Extended lymph-node dissection for gastric cancer. N Engl J Med 1999;340(12):908–14.

[64] Cuschieri AF, Fayers P, Fielding J, et al. Post-operative morbidity and mortality after D1 and D2 resections for gastric cancer: preliminary results of the MRC rabdomised controlled surgical trial. Lancet 1996;347:995–9.

[65] Brady MS, Rogatko A, Dent LL, et al. Effect of splenectomy on morbidity and survival following curative gastrectomy for carcinoma. Arch Surg 1991;126:359–64.

[66] Kitamura K, Nishida S, Ichikawa D, et al. No survival benefit from combined pancreaticosplenectomy and total gastrectomy for gastric cancer. Br J Surg 1999;86:119–22.

[67] Lee KY, Noh SH, Hyung WJ, et al. Impact of splenectomy for lymph node dissection on long-term surgical outcome in gastric cancer. Ann Surg Oncol 2001;8(5):402–6.

[68] Csendes A, Burdiles P, Rojas J, et al. A prospective randomized study comparing D2 total gastrectomy versus D2 total gastrectomy plus splenectomy in 187 patients with gastric carcinoma. Surgery 2002;131(4):401–7.

[69] Bando E, Yonemura Y, Taniguchi K, et al. Outcome of ratio of lymph node metastasis in gastric carcinoma. Ann Surg Oncol 2002;9(8):775–84.

[70] Liu KJ, Loewen M, Atten MJ, et al. The survival of stage III gastric cancer patients is affected by the number of lymph nodes removed. Surgery 2003;134(4):639–44.

[71] Karpeh MS, Leon L, Klimstra D, et al. Lymph node staging in gastric cancer: is location more important than number? an analysis of 1,038 patients. Ann Surg 2000;232(3):362–71.

[72] Volpe CM, Driscoll DL, Douglass HO. Outcome of patients with proximal gastric cancer depends on the extent of resection and number of resected lymph nodes. Ann Surg Oncol 2000;7(2):139–44.

[73] Greene FL, Page DL, Fleming ID, et al. AJCC Cancer staging manual. 6th edition. New York: Springer-Verlag; 2002. p. 99.

[74] Furukawa H, Hiratsuka M, Imaoka S, et al. Phase II study of limited surgery for early gastric cancer: segmental gastric resection. Ann Surg Oncol 1999;6(2):166–70.

[75] Yokota T, Ishiyama S, Saito T, et al. Treatment strategy of limited surgery in the treatment guidelines for gastric cancer in Japan. Lancet Oncol 2003;4(7):423–8.

[76] Hochwald SN, Brennan MF, Klimstra DS, et al. Is lymphadenectomy necessary for early gastric cancer? Ann Surg Oncol 1999;6(7):664–70.

ELSEVIER
SAUNDERS

Surg Oncol Clin N Am
14 (2005) 533–552

SURGICAL
ONCOLOGY CLINICS
OF NORTH AMERICA

Pancreaticoduodenectomy (Whipple operation)

Thomas E. Clancy, MD[a,b],
Stanley W. Ashley, MD[a,b,*]

[a]Department of Surgery, Brigham and Women's Hospital,
75 Francis Street, Boston, MA 02115, USA
[b]Harvard Medical School, 25 Shattuck Street, Boston, MA 02115, USA

Surgical resection is the only potentially curative therapy for pancreatic and periampullary tumors. Pancreaticoduodenectomy, the most common operation performed for these neoplasms, is one of the most specialized and challenging procedures performed by gastrointestinal surgeons. With a century of progress in surgical technique and postsurgical care, previous perioperative mortality rates of 20% to 30% have fallen to less than 5%. Unfortunately, improvements in early mortality have been associated with only modest improvements in long-term survival because most patients suffer from early locoregional recurrence or distant metastases, even after undergoing curative resection. In the last decade, the use of data from large series and prospective clinical trials has allowed greater standardization of the techniques used in pancreaticoduodenectomy, although numerous controversial issues remain. This article reviews the early history of pancreatic resection for cancer, the refinement of surgical technique over the subsequent decades, and the current status of pancreaticoduodenectomy.

Early pancreatic resections for cancer

Although a few attempts at pancreatic resection for cancer were described as early as the late 1800s, surgeons at that time encountered formidable challenges to routine pancreatic surgery. Anatomic constraints frustrated easy surgical access and hampered accurate and early diagnosis of pancreatic cancer. Furthermore, a full understanding of pancreatic physiology and the

* Corresponding author. Department of Surgery, Brigham and Women's Hospital, 75 Francis Street, Boston, MA 02115.
  E-mail address: sashley@partners.org (S.W. Ashley).

1055-3207/05/$ - see front matter © 2005 Elsevier Inc. All rights reserved.
doi:10.1016/j.soc.2005.05.006

physiologic consequences of pancreatic resection was lacking at the time [1]. Surgeons who experimented with the procedure found inherent difficulties particularly in the surgery of the pancreatic head, including a loss of pancreatic function and the interruption of blood flow to the duodenum [2]. Trendelenburg may have performed the first pancreatic resection when he resected a spindle cell sarcoma of the pancreatic tail in 1882, although the patient died the following day [3]. Aside from isolated reports of pancreatic tumor resection by Billroth in 1884 [2], Ruggi in 1889 [4], and Briggs in 1890 [5], routine pancreatic resection was still decades away.

Skepticism felt by surgeons of the day was reflected by VonMickulicz-Radecki [6], who wrote in 1903 that the pancreas has "no clinical interest, as it was almost impossible for the surgeon to reach it." Similarly, Moynihan's chapter in the 1906 edition of his book "Abdominal Operations" [7] states that "the treatment of malignant disease of the pancreas by the surgeon can hardly be said to exist...the mechanical difficulties of the operation are well-nigh insuperable, and that if boldness and good fortune are the operators gifts, the result to the patient hardly justifies the means." In the absence of resection, techniques were developed for palliation for obstructing pancreatic tumors. Cholecystogastrostomy for biliary diversion, popularized by Terrier [8] and Jaboulay [9], was combined with gastroenterostomy for gastric decompression. These methods were later used to restore gastrointestinal continuity after pancreatic resection [10].

The persistent efforts of early surgical investigators, coupled with an improved understanding of anatomy and physiology, soon led to success with limited pancreatic resection. In the late 1800s, surgeons such as MacBurney [11] and Kocher [12] described elective duodenotomy and papillotomy to extract biliary stones. This technique was soon used thereafter by Halsted [13] at Johns Hopkins Hospital, in 1898, to perform a transduodenal ampullary resection, perhaps the first successful resection described for a periampullary neoplasm. Similar reports by Mayo [14], Hartmann and Navarro [15], Kausch [16], and others followed in succession. Other contemporary advances included the description by Kocher, in 1903, of extensive duodenal mobilization and the description by Kocher's apprentice, Cesar Roux [17], of the Roux-en-Y procedure, later used in cholecystojejunostomy and hepaticojejunostomy.

The Whipple procedure

Resection of the pancreatic head remains a formidable technical challenge, usually requiring removal of not only a major portion of the pancreas but also the distal bile duct and duodenum, which requires multiple anastomoses for reconstruction. Numerous technical variations have been and continue to be described (Fig. 1). The first true pancreaticoduodenectomy for a pancreatic head lesion was described by Codivilla, in 1898. The duodenum, pancreatic head, and pylorus were resected, the common bile

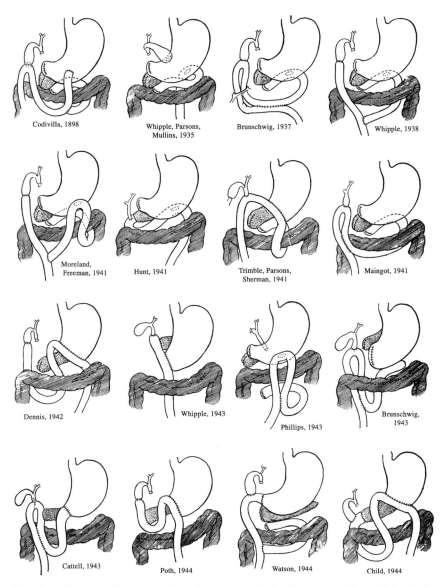

Fig. 1. Techniques of reconstruction after pancreaticoduodenectomy. (*From* Maingot R. Pancreatic tumors. In: Abdominal operations. 4th edition. New York: Appleton Century Crofts; 1961. p. 563–603; with permission.)

duct was ligated above the pancreas, with subsequent cholecystojejunostomy, and Roux-en-Y gastroenterostomy was performed. The patient survived only 21 days. Of note, no efforts were made to control the pancreatic fistula, perhaps because of an incomplete appreciation of the physiology of pancreatic secretion. Reports of the procedure and the subsequent postoperative course noted that "a serous appearing liquid leaked continuously from the wound...abundant diarrheal episodes of unused material" [1]. VonMickulicz-Radecki [6] later argued that pancreatic secretions were not benign and should be kept from the abdominal cavity if at all possible. To prevent the digestion of retroperitoneal fat, Coffey [18] described a method of pancreatic drainage through an anastomosis between the pancreatic tail and a loop of small intestine. It was Kausch [19], an apprentice of VonMickulicz-Radecki, who, in 1909, used the technique of pancreaticoenterostomy to perform the first successful pancreaticoduodenectomy. This was a two-stage procedure in which a cholecystojejunostomy preceded resection by 6 weeks [1,19]. Biliary drainage was performed to minimize complications of jaundice, including bleeding, which was exacerbated by vitamin K malabsorption in the jaundiced patient. In the second stage of the procedure, a gastrojejunostomy was performed, with resection of the first and second portions of the duodenum and anastomosis of the third portion of the duodenum to the pancreatic remnant. Other surgeons repeated this two-stage procedure [20,21] over the subsequent 2 decades.

The landmark 1935 publication of Whipple, Parsons, and Mullins [22] reported on the management of 80 cases of ampullary carcinoma, including transduodenal excision, duodenectomy, resection of the common duct, and two-stage resection of the pancreas and duodenum. Their description of pancreaticoduodenectomy entailed an initial stage of posterior gastroenterostomy, ligation and division of the common bile duct, and cholecystogastrostomy for biliary drainage (Fig. 2). A second stage performed 4 weeks later consisted of a duodenal resection with a wedge of the pancreatic head and ampulla, with oversewing of the pancreatic stump, and the placement of drains. Unlike the procedure by Kausch before them, Whipple and colleagues did not drain pancreatic secretions with a pancreaticojejunostomy; of note, neither did Whipple and colleagues perform a gastric resection, thus sparing the pylorus [23]. Although Whipple was not the first to describe the procedure, his significant contributions to the field have resulted in his name being virtually synonymous with the procedure of pancreaticoduodenectomy.

The operation described by Whipple and colleagues underwent many early modifications. Early challenges included a desire to modify the biliary-enteric anastomosis to reduce intestinal reflux. Hunt [24] has described a number of variations, including cholecystoduodenostomy, choledochogastrostomy, cholecystojejunostomy, and choledochojejunostomy. Both Hunt [24] and Brunschwig [25] also have described the use of Roux's Y-shaped enteroenterostomy to limit enteric reflux into the bile duct. The subsequent discovery of vitamin K enabled surgeons to overcome the difficulty of coagulopathy in jaundiced patients, and therefore, the two-stage procedure with initial biliary bypass became unnecessary. A partial gastrectomy procedure was added by Trimble and colleagues [26], who

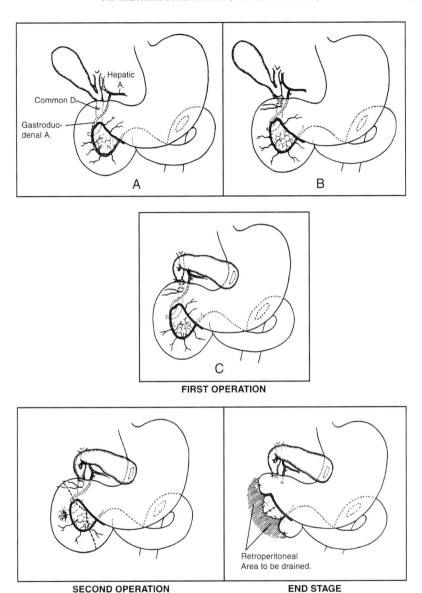

Fig. 2. Two-stage pancreaticoduodenectomy, as popularized originally by Whipple. (*From* Whipple AO, Parsons N, Mullins C. Treatment of carcinoma of the ampulla of Vater. Ann Surg 1935;102:763–79; with permission.)

concurrently with Whipple [27], described a one-stage pancreaticoduodenectomy. By 1942, the "Whipple procedure" was described as initial vitamin K therapy, surgical resection of the distal stomach, the entire duodenum, the terminal common bile duct, and the head of the pancreas, and the reestablishment of continuity by means of a choledochojejunostomy, pancreaticojejunostomy, and gastrojejunostomy (Fig. 3).

Despite these early technical advances, the operative mortality for pancreaticoduodenectomy remained considerable, as high as 20% to 30% [28]. Survival rates reported for all patients with pancreatic cancer remained dismal, with 5-year survival rates of less than 5%. Only approximately 10% of patients who underwent surgery for pancreatic cancer were deemed appropriate for the procedure, and, of those who underwent resection, fewer than 13% would survive 5 years [29]. Several authors suggested that, even for resectable pancreatic cancer, palliative surgical bypass produced outcomes comparable to or better than pancreaticoduodenectomy [30]. With decades of refinement in technique and concentration of experience, operative mortality gradually decreased to a modern standard of less than 5% (Table 1) [31–46]. Furthermore, surgical modifications were developed in an attempt to increase oncologic benefit (total pancreatectomy and regional pancreatectomy) and to limit complications (pylorus-sparing pancreaticoduodenectomy) [47,48].

Total pancreatectomy

Cattell and Pyrtek [49] have described a series of patients treated with pancreaticoduodenectomy at the Lahey Clinic in Boston, in 1949, in whom the mortality rate for resection for pancreatic carcinoma (17%) greatly exceeded that for ampullary carcinoma (5%). Postulating the dissemination of cancer cells during transection of an obstructed pancreatic duct, the

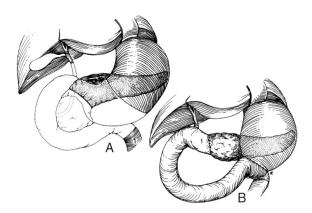

Fig. 3. Today's standard pancreaticoduodenectomy procedure. (*A*) The areas removed include the distal stomach, duodenum, pancreatic head, distal bile duct, and gallbladder. (*B*) One-stage reconstruction with pancreaticojejunostomy, choledochojejunostomy, and gastrojejunostomy. (*From* Ashley SW, Reber HA. Cancer and other neoplastic disorders of the exocrine pancreas. In: Gitnick G, editor. Principles and practice of gastroenterology and hepatology. 2nd edition. New York: Elsevier; 1994. p. 501–10.)

Table 1
Selected series of pancreaticoduodenectomy: perioperative morbidity and mortality and long-term survival

Study	Study period	N	30-d mortality (%)	Total morbidity (%)	Pancreatic. leakage (%)	5-yr survival Pancreatic CA	Ampullary CA	Bile duct CA
Smith (1973) [31]	1946–1972	224	8			6	35	19
Warren et al (1975) [32]	1942–1971	139	11		7	13	32	25
Tepper et al (1976) [33]	1963–1973	31	16			15		
Nakase et al (1977) [34]	1949–1974	824	21	49	14	3	6	3
Cooperman et al (1981) [35]	1940–1978	92	14		37	11	26	22
Herter et al (1982) [36]	1940–1978	102	15	58	9	7	28	33
Lerut et al [37]	1967–1981	103	11	20	15	≤1	50	
Grace et al (1986) [38]	1975–1984	96	6	39	24	3	62	52
Crist et al (1987) [39]	1969–1986	88	12	47		18		
Trede et al (1990) [40]	1985–1989	118		18		24		
Geer and Brennan (1993) [41]	1983–1990	799	5		2	24		
Nitecki et al (1993) [42]	1981–1991	186	3	32		7		
Tsao et al (1994) [43]	1979–1992	106	2	39	14	7	45	33
Yeo et al (1995) [44]	1970–1994	201	5			21		
Fernandez et al (1995) [45]	1991–1994	142	0	43	6			
Yeo et al (1997) [46]	1990–1996	650	1.4	41	14	20	32	10

Several large series of pancreaticoduodenectomy from the past four decades are presented to demonstrate general trends. No claim is made regarding completeness. Mortality and survival rates are difficult to compare between studies given different surgical indications between studies. Morbidity data are difficult to compare given differences in reporting practices for complications.

Abbreviation: CA, cancer.

authors suggested that "the employment of total pancreatectomy in early carcinoma of the head of the pancreas offers the only chance of possible improvement of these results [1]." The procedure also obviated the need for pancreaticojejunostomy, at that time the major source of morbidity with the procedure. Collins and coworkers [50], from the Peter Bent Brigham Hospital in Boston, argued that three possible explanations existed for the persistence or recurrence of pancreatic cancer after partial pancreatectomy: micrometastatic spread, de novo development of cancer in the pancreatic remnant, or microscopic spread of cancer throughout the pancreas with positive resection margins. Of these, two explanations would be solved potentially by total pancreatectomy. Early reports by Rockey in 1943 [51] and Ross in 1954 [52] drew some attention to total pancreatectomy for cancer. Although early series have reported an operative mortality rate of 37% [53], the appropriate use of insulin and pancreatic enzymes allowed control of the diabetic state and malnutrition after total pancreatectomy. Furthermore, a major source of perioperative morbidity was avoided by eliminating the need for a pancreaticojejunal anastomosis. Total pancreatectomy was therefore recommended by some surgeons to treat the high incidence of nonpalpable tumor extension into the pancreatic body and new tumor development in the pancreatic remnant [50].

Subsequent work by these authors confirmed the frequency of microscopic positive margins after the Whipple procedure. A 1979 review from Peter Bent Brigham Hospital has demonstrated that 36% of patients with carcinoma of the pancreatic head had synchronous disease in the body and tail. The identification of multicentric disease of the pancreas has led some authors to question whether standard pancreaticoduodenectomy is a sufficient oncologic operation [54,55]. Brooks and colleagues [56] have presented a series of 48 patients who underwent total pancreatectomy for pancreatic cancer over a period of 16 years. Although the mortality rate was 18% in the first 6 years, with improvements in perioperative care there were no hospital deaths in the final 28 cases, with a 5-year survival of 14%. Other investigators simultaneously reported improvements in morbidity and mortality after the Whipple procedure [39], and despite the problem of multicentricity of pancreatic tumors, overall long-term survival was similar after standard pancreaticoduodenectomy or total pancreatectomy. Without a demonstration of improved outcomes and with the added morbidity of fragile diabetes, total pancreatectomy did not, therefore, achieve routine use in curative surgery for pancreatic cancer.

Regional pancreatectomy: early reports and vascular resection

In most early series, only approximately 10% of patients who underwent exploratory surgery for pancreatic cancer had disease that was amenable to resection. The unique anatomic constraints facing the pancreatic surgeon were identified by McDermott [57], who stated, in 1952, that "the standard pancreatoduodenal resection is so limited in scope by the location of the portal system of veins that, not only is the resectability rate discouragingly low (20% in our series), but no adequate block dissection has been possible." Whether pancreaticoduodenectomy or total pancreatectomy was performed for pancreatic cancer, over 50% of patients were found with local recurrence in the resection bed in some reports [33]. In an attempt to improve local control, Fortner [58] built on the technique by Child and colleagues' [28] portal vein resection and described the technique of regional pancreatectomy. This procedure added a regional lymphadenectomy and portal vein resection to the standard Whipple operation, aiming to improve disease control by extirpating all regional tissues that might harbor residual cancer cells. In addition to potentially improving disease control compared with conventional resection, it was suggested that regional pancreatectomy might allow for the resection of large lesions considered previously to be unsuitable for surgery.

Early small series with regional pancreatectomy have demonstrated conflicting results. Although some series have demonstrated comparable morbidity and mortality rates with regional pancreatectomy compared with the Whipple procedure [59], other investigators have described increased morbidity and technical difficulty with negligible survival benefit. In a 1989 series from the National Cancer Institute, Sindelar [60] has described a 55% complication rate and perioperative mortality of 20% in 20 patients who underwent regional pancreatectomy. Other series have describe a survival benefit from regional pancreatectomy [61,62]. The high rate of morbidity and mortality associated with this procedure, resulting particularly from arterial reconstruction, and a lack of universally demonstrated survival benefit, prevented widespread acceptance of Fortner's technique.

Using a modified regional pancreatectomy limited to the resection of the involved portal or superior mesenteric veins without radical lymphadenectomy, modern surgeons have demonstrated excellent results. The published experience from the M.D. Anderson Cancer Center and Memorial Sloan-Kettering Cancer Center [63–65] suggests that isolated tumor adherence or invasion of the superior mesenteric vein or portal vein is not a contraindication to resection. It is believed that tumor involvement of the superior mesenteric artery or celiac axis usually includes involvement of the mesenteric neural plexus, making negative excision margins nearly impossible to achieve [66]. However, venous involvement at the superior mesenteric-portal vein confluence without arterial involvement is believed to be a function of tumor location and not a marker of aggressiveness [64,67]. Positive surgical margins with tumor left on the lateral wall of the vein are known to result in a survival duration similar to locally advanced disease that has been treated nonsurgically [68]. Patients with isolated vein involvement without tumor extension to the superior mesenteric artery or celiac axis have therefore been considered for en-bloc venous resection and reconstruction [69].

Brennan and colleagues [63] have shown that most patients who require portal vein resection may undergo reconstruction with a primary end-to-end anastomosis and that vein resection may be performed with a resulting rate of morbidity similar to pancreatic resections without portal venous reconstruction. Others authors have reported superior results with internal jugular vein interpositional grafts to avoid splenic vein compromise and left-sided portal hypertension [65]. Preoperative contrast-enhanced CT scanning has been shown to predict the need for superior mesenteric or portal veins in 84% of patients [65]; and the sensitivity of endoscopic ultrasonography for venous involvement has been reported as ranging from 43% to 62%, with a specificity of 79% to 91% [70].

Regional pancreatectomy: extended lymphadenectomy

The involvement of peripancreatic lymph nodes with metastatic pancreatic cancer is known to be associated with a poor prognosis. As noted above, Fortner [58], in 1973. suggested that resectability and outcomes for pancreatic cancer patients may be improved by regional pancreatectomy, including venous reconstruction and wide retroperitoneal soft tissue dissection. However, whether the removal of all positive lymph nodes improves survival has continued to be controversial. Several retrospective series from Japan have reported improved 5-year survival rates after pancreaticoduodenectomy with extended lymph node dissection [71,72].

Recently, two randomized clinical trials of extended lymphadenectomy in patients with pancreatic adenocarcinoma have been performed [73,74]. These two studies randomized 81 and 294 patients, respectively, to either standard lymphadenectomy, including the peripancreatic nodes, or extended lymphadenectomy. The precise degree of lymphadenectomy did vary between studies. In the study by Pedrazzoli and colleagues [73], extended lymphadenectomy included the removal of lymph nodes along the aorta from the diaphragm to the inferior mesenteric artery, from the hepatic hilum and both renal hila, and along the celiac trunk and superior mesenteric artery. In the study by Yeo and coworkers [74], a pylorus-preserving technique was used in the standard dissection, which added a distal gastrectomy plus retroperitoneal lymphadenectomy to the extended procedure, but clearance of the superior mesenteric, celiac, or common hepatic arteries was not performed. Of note, extended lymphadenectomy did not increase morbidity in either study, and the overall survival rate did not differ in either study. In the study by Pedrazzoli [73], a post-hoc analysis of patient subgroups suggests a significantly longer survival rate after extended lymphadenectomy when analysis is limited to node-positive patients. The Yeo group [74], however, did not note any statistical difference in survival with the more extensive procedure.

Several authors have pointed out the difficulty in demonstrating a statistically valid difference with extended lymphadenectomy in the context of a clinical trial. Pisters and colleagues [69] have argued that extended lymphadenectomy potentially will confer a benefit only in limited circumstances: an R0 resection must be achieved (50%–80% of cases), the second-echelon or N2 nodes must be positive (10%–15% of cases), and positive N2 nodes must occur in the absence of visceral metastases (true N2 M0 cases are estimated to occur in only 5% of positive N2 nodes). Using these estimates, only approximately 0.4% of patients would potentially benefit from an extended lymphadenectomy with pancreatic resection, requiring an enormous sample size and long accrual time for a properly powered study. Existing studies document the relative safety of extended lymphadenectomy, and Nguyen and colleagues [75] have documented no differences in long-term quality of life between standard and radical resection. Still, the lack of convincing data supporting a survival benefit to radical lymph node dissection has led most authors to abandon it as a part of routine pancreatic cancer surgery.

Pylorus-preserving pancreaticoduodenectomy

Whipple's description of the two-stage pancreaticoduodenectomy involved preserving the entire stomach, with the pylorus left as a blind stump. To avoid leakage from the blind stump, the procedure was later revised to remove the pylorus and distal stomach [26]. The preservation of these structures was later performed in an effort to decrease surgical morbidity. Traverso and Longmire [76] reintroduced pylorus preservation to the operation in 1978 (Fig. 4), originally to reduce the incidence of marginal ulceration at the gastroenterostomy, and the procedure subsequently became a standard in some centers [46]. Pylorus-preserving pancreaticoduodenectomy (PPPD) has been compared with the standard pancreaticoduodenectomy with partial gastrectomy (Whipple operation) in terms of nutritional status, oncologic adequacy, morbidity and mortality, and other factors [77]. Survival rates after PPPD have compared favorably with those of the classic Whipple resection [78], and most authors agree that PPPD does not impair the achievement of appropriate surgical margins unless tumors are located on the anterosuperior surface of the pancreatic head, close to the pylorus [77]. Perioperative morbidity has been shown to be similar whether or not the pylorus is preserved [79–81]. Some authors have suggested that PPPD may be complicated by delayed gastric emptying [82,83], although others have not documented this problem [84,85]. Still other investigators have argued that stomach preservation allows improved long-term gastrointestinal function, avoiding such difficulties as dumping, diarrhea, dyspeptic complaints, and gastrojejunal anastomotic ulcers. Furthermore, nutritional status and weight gain have been reported by some authors to be significantly improved in patients who have undergone PPPD versus those who have undergone the conventional Whipple procedure [80,86].

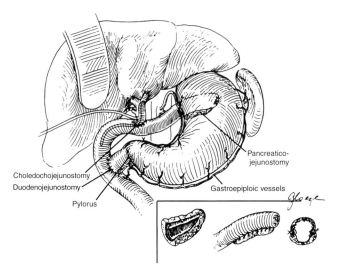

Fig. 4. Pylorus-preserving pancreaticoduodenectomy, as described originally by Traverso and Longmire, with the technique for pancreaticojejunostomy (*inset*). (*From* Traverso LW, Longmire WP Jr. Preservation of the pylorus in pancreaticoduodenectomy. J Am Coll Surg (Surg Gynecol Obstet) 1978;146:959–62; with permission.)

Although most studies that have compared outcomes from conventional pancreaticoduodenectomy with those from PPPD have been retrospective and nonrandomized, three recent randomized, controlled trials of PPPD versus Whipple for periampullary cancer have been reported [87–89]. Although one study [87] has shown no difference between perioperative morbidity and mortality and a trend toward greater delayed gastric emptying after pylorus preservation, a second study [88] has suggested higher morbidity with the classic Whipple procedure and no differences in gastric emptying. With only 31 and 77 patients, respectively, each study was underpowered to definitively address the safety and outcomes of these two procedures. In a larger, prospective multicenter study, Tran and associates [89] analyzed 170 patients with pancreatic or periampullary neoplasms randomized to PPPD versus the standard Whipple procedure. No differences in operative time or blood loss, delayed gastric emptying, operative mortality, or survival between the two techniques were found. Although surgeon and institutional biases remain, the existing evidence does not support the superiority of either procedure.

Pancreaticoenterostomy

Given the considerable morbidity resulting from a pancreatic fistula, many technical modifications of pancreaticoenterostomy have been proposed, including pancreaticojejunostomy versus pancreaticogastrostomy. In a prospective trial from Johns Hopkins Hospital [44], these two methods were compared using a two-layer pancreaticoenteric anastomosis. Of note, the incidence of anastomotic leak was virtually identical for the two procedures (11% for pancreaticojejunostomy and 12% for pancreaticogastrostomy). This well-powered study demonstrates the virtual equivalence in morbidity and mortality rates for the two methods of pancreatic anastomosis. Other studies have examined different techniques of pancreaticojejunostomy; for example, an end-to-end invaginating technique has been compared with an end-to-side, duct-to-mucosa technique, with a stent [90]. Of note, there was a nonsignificant trend toward higher morbidity with end-to-end anastomosis, as well as a trend toward a higher pancreatic fistulae rate with the end-to-end technique (15% versus 4%). Bassi and colleagues [91] recently completed a prospective study in which 144 patients were randomly assigned to a duct-to-mucosa pancreaticojejunostomy or a one-layer end-to-side pancreaticojejunostomy. The outcomes showed virtually no difference in the rate of pancreatic fistula, which was 14% and 13% in the two arms. In summary, good randomized evidence suggests that pancreaticogastrostomy and pancreaticojejunostomy have equivalent complications, as do different methods of pancreaticojejunostomy.

Pancreaticoduodenectomy: modern series

A brief examination of surgical series of pancreaticoduodenectomies demonstrates a recent decline in perioperative mortality. A selection of series published in the last 40 years is listed in Table 1. Yeo and colleagues [46] have recently described a series of 650 pancreaticoduodenectomies from a single institution. These results have set new standards for outcomes after this operation. An operative mortality rate (inhospital or within 30 days) of 1.4% was reported, a considerable improvement over the 20% to 30% operative mortality reported earlier [10]. The postoperative complication rate of 41% included 19% of patients with delayed gastric emptying, 14% with pancreatic fistula, and 10% with wound infection. The decline in perioperative mortality is likely multifactorial. Improvements in critical care, nutritional support, radiologic services, management of complications and systemic comorbidities, and increased single-institution experience are likely all related to improved perioperative outcomes.

This Hopkins group [92] also has reported actual 5-year survival data on patients who underwent periampullary adenocarcinoma. The median survival after resection was 12 months, with an actual 5-year survival rate of 15%. As many as 72% of patients had nodal involvement, and 31% had positive resection margins, usually at the level of the hepatic or superior mesenteric arteries. Although these results are sobering, the data suggest modest improvements in survival compared with earlier series. For instance, a 1987 review of over 50 case series has suggested that the 5-year survival rate after resection for pancreatic adenocarcinoma is approximately 4% [93]. The reason for improved outcomes is unclear, but possibilities include improved patient selection, operative technique, and improvements in adjuvant therapy. Improved outcomes are seen especially in selected subgroups of patients and may not be representative of all "resectable" patients. Whether the published long-term survival rates of approximately 20% represent a true increase in survival or an artifact of patient selection may remain a matter of debate, and long-term survival for pancreatic cancer in particular remains poor. Still, resection remains the only chance for cure for periampullary carcinoma.

Volume outcome

Significant attention has focused on whether certain high-risk surgical procedures should be regionalized to high-volume centers and high-volume surgeons. A number of studies have demonstrated convincingly that short-term outcomes for pancreaticoduodenectomy are significantly better at hospitals where a higher volume of the procedures is performed. A selection of series comparing perioperative mortality in low- and high-volume hospitals is shown in Table 2 [94–103]. The mechanisms behind these findings also have been the subject of some debate. Undoubtedly, systems of care and nonsurgical medical personnel, including critical care physicians, anesthesiologists, radiologists, and nurses, may contribute heavily to the observed effect. In fact, a relationship between perioperative mortality after pancreaticoduodenectomy and the volume of nonpancreatic high-risk procedures has been demonstrated [104]. This suggests that mortality after pancreaticoduodenectomy is not related solely to institutional experience with this procedure but also may be related to the general systems of care for high-risk patients present at tertiary institutions and high-volume referral centers. Sosa and colleagues [97] suggest that the individual surgeon volume is less important than such systems of care. In contrast, Birkmeyer and colleagues [105] suggest that the individual surgeon volume accounts for as much as 50% of the observed effect of hospital volume; in other words, high-volume hospitals demonstrate better outcomes in part because patients are more likely to be treated by high-volume surgeons. Little consensus exists on how these data might be used to distribute patient volume or resources. However, these studies present an ongoing opportunity to identify the optimal surgical and perioperative practices of high-volume surgeons and hospitals that contribute to improved outcomes.

Future trends in pancreatic surgery

Surgical resection remains the only hope for cure for periampullary cancer. Although decades of refinement have significantly reduced the

Table 2
Selected series comparing perioperative mortality after pancreaticoduodenectomy in low-volume versus high-volume hospitals

Study	Study period	Overall mortality (%)	Mortality at low-volume hospitals (%) (criteria: cases/y)	Mortality at high-volume hospitals (%) (criteria: cases/y)	P value
Lieberman et al (1995) [94]	1984–1991	12.9	18.9 ($<2/y$)	5.5 ($>10/y$)	≤.001
Gordon et al (1995) [95]	1988–1993	7.7	19.1 (1–5/y)	2.2 ($>20/y$)	≤.001
Glasgow and Mulvihill (1996) [96]	1990–1994	9.9	14.1 (1–5/y)	3.5 ($>50/y$)	N/A
Sosa et al (1998) [97]	1990–1995	N/A	19 ($\leq5/y$)	1 ($>20/y$)	≤.001
Birkmeyer et al (1999) [98]	1992–1995	11.1	16.1 ($\leq1/y$)	4.1 ($>5/y$)	≤.001
Begg et al (1998) [99]	1984–1993	N/A	12.9 ($\leq5/y$)	5.8 ($>11/y$)	≤.004
Simunovic et al (1999) [100]	1988–1995	9.7	11.3 ($\leq3/y$)	3.4 ($>6/y$)	≤.01
Kingsnorth (2000) [101]	1992–1995	N/A	16 ($\leq1/y$)	4 ($>5/y$)	≤.001
Birkmeyer et al (2002) [102]	1994–1999	N/A	16.3 ($\leq1/y$)	3.8 ($>16/y$)	N/A
Ho and Heslin (2003) [103]	1988–1998	9.5	9.5–15.9 (1–3/y)	3.3–4.7 ($>10/y$)	N/A

Several series are shown that have examined the relationship between hospital volume of pancreaticoduodenectomy and surgical outcomes. Criteria for classifying an institutional low-volume versus a high volume vary in the literature and are individually defined for the studies above.

Abbreviation: NA, not applicable.

perioperative morbidity and mortality of pancreatic resection, long-term survival is poor. Surgeons in the future will continue to be challenged by the underlying biology of periampullary malignancies, and progress will depend largely on an improved understanding of the molecular mechanisms underlying carcinogenesis. The identification of premalignant changes in the pancreas (pancreatic intraepithelial neoplasia) has suggested that pancreatic cancer occurs with the gradual accumulation of genetic aberrations in epithelial cells, from low- to high-grade dysplasia and frank malignancy [106]. Novel biomarkers might serve as the means of screening or early diagnosis and thereby increased resectability. The identification of molecular markers of prognosis may allow molecular profiling of tumors for prognosis and for the early identification of which patients would benefit from resection. In addition, novel therapeutic targets remain potentially undiscovered. Undoubtedly, future progress in pancreatic cancer surgery will be closely related to research into the underlying biology of this disease.

References

[1] McClusky DA III, Skandalakis LJ, Colborn GL, et al. Harbinger or hermit? pancreatic anatomy and surgery through the ages: part 2. World J Surg 2002;26:1370–81.

[2] Senn N. Experimental surgery. Chicago: WT Keener; 1889.

[3] Brunschwig A. The surgery of pancreatic tumors. St. Louis: CV Mosby; 1942.

[4] Ruggi GF. Intorno ad un caso di carcinoma primitivo del pancreas, curato e guarito con l'asportazione del tumore. Giornale Internazionale della Scienza Medica 1890;12:81–5 [in Italian].

[5] Briggs E. Tumor of the pancreas, laparotomy, recovery. Medical and Surgical Journal 1890;58:154–69.

[6] VonMickulicz-Radecki J. Surgery of the pancreas. Ann Surg 1903;38:1–9.

[7] Moynihan B. Neoplasms of the pancreas. In: Moynihan B, editor. Abdominal operations. Philadelphia: WB Saunders; 1906.

[8] Terrier F. Remarques sur 2 cas, l'un de cholecystoduodenostomie, l'autre de cholecysto-gastrostomie. Rev Chir 1896;16:169–78 [in French].

[9] Jaboulay M. La cholecystogastrostomie pour les tumeurs de la tete du pancreas. Lyon Med 1898;89:365–74 [in French].

[10] Praderi RC, editor. History of pancreatic surgery. New York: Churchill Livingstone; 1993.

[11] MacBurney CH. Removal of biliare calculi from the common duct by the duodenal route. Ann Surg 1878;28:481–91.

[12] Kocher T. Ein fall von choledocho-duodenostomia interna wegen gallenstein. Korrespondenzbl Sweitz Artze 1895;1:192–9 [in German].

[13] Halstead W. Contributions to the surgery of the bile passages, especially of the common bile-duct. Boston Medical and Surgical Journal 1899;141:645–61.

[14] Mayo W. Cancer of the common bile duct: report of a case of carcinoma of the duodenal end of the common duct with successful excision. St Paul Medical Journal 1901;3:374–85.

[15] Hartmann H, Navarro A. Cancere de l'ampoule de Vater: extirpation guerison. Bull Mem Soc Chir Paris 1910;2:1340–5 [in French].

[16] Kausch W. Das carcinom der papilla duodeni und seine radikale entfernung. Beitrage zur Klinishen Chirurgie 1912;78:29–33 [in German].

[17] Roux C. De la gastro-enterostomie. Revue de Gynecologie et Chirurgie Abdominale 1897; 1:67–81 [in French].

[18] Coffey R. Pancreatico-enterostomy and pancreatectomy: a preliminary report. Ann Surg 1909;50:1238–43.

[19] Kausch W. Die Resektion des mittleren duodenus: eine typische operation: vorlaufige mitteilung. Zentralblatt fur Chirurgie 1909;39 [in German].

[20] Tenani O. Contributo alla chirurgia della papilla di Vater. Policlinico 1922;29:291–8 [in Italian].

[21] Hirschel G. Die Resektion des duodenums mit der papille wegen cephalique. Rev Chir Orthop Reparatrice Appar Mot 1914;61:1728–41 [in German].

[22] Whipple AO, Parsons N, Mullins C. Treatment of carcinoma of the ampulla of Vater. Ann Surg 1935;102:763–79.

[23] Peters JH, Carey LC. Historical review of pancreaticoduodenectomy. Am J Surg 1991;161: 219–25.

[24] Hunt VC. Surgical management of carcinoma of the ampulla of Vater and of the periampullary portion of the duodenum. Ann Surg 1941;114:570–602.

[25] Brunschwig A. Resection of the head of pancreas and duodenum for carcinoma-pancreatoduodenectomy. J Am Coll Surg (Surg Gynecol Obstet) 1937;65:681–9.

[26] Trimble IR, Parsons JW, Sherman CP. A one-stage operation for the cure of carcinoma of the ampulla of Vater and of the head of the pancreas. J Am Coll Surg (Surg Gynecol Obstet) 1941;73:711–9.

[27] Whipple AO. The rationale of radical surgery for cancer of the pancreas and ampullary region. Ann Surg 1941;114:612–23.

[28] Child CG III, Holswade GR, McClure RD Jr, et al. Pancreaticoduodenectomy with resection of the portal vein in the *Macaca mulatta* monkey and in man. J Am Coll Surg (Surg Gynecol Obstet) 1952;94:31–45.

[29] Rhoads JE, Zintel HA, Helwig J Jr. Results of operations of the Whipple type in pancreaticoduodenal carcinoma. Ann Surg 1957;146:661–5.

[30] Crile G Jr. The advantages of bypass operations over radical pancreatoduodenectomy in the treatment of pancreatic carcinoma. J Am Coll Surg (Surg Gynecol Obstet) 1970;130: 1049–53.

[31] Smith R. Progress in the surgical treatment of pancreatic disease. Am J Surg 1973;125: 143–53.

[32] Warren KW, Choe DS, Plaza J, et al. Results of radical resection for periampullary cancer. Ann Surg 1975;181:534–40.

[33] Tepper J, Nardi G, Sutt H. Carcinoma of the pancreas: review of MGH experience from 1963 to 1973: analysis of surgical failure and implications for radiation therapy. Cancer 1976;37:1519–24.

[34] Nakase A, Matsumoto Y, Uchida K, et al. Surgical treatment of cancer of the pancreas and the periampullary region: cumulative results in 57 institutions in Japan. Ann Surg 1977; 185:52–7.

[35] Cooperman AM, Herter FP, Marboe CA, et al. Pancreatoduodenal resection and total pancreatectomy: an institutional review. Surgery 1981;90:707–12.

[36] Herter FP, Cooperman AM, Ahlborn TN, et al. Surgical experience with pancreatic and periampullary cancer. Ann Surg 1982;195:274–81.

[37] Lerut JP, Gianello PR, Otte JB, et al. Pancreaticoduodenal resection: surgical experience and evaluation of risk factors in 103 patients. Ann Surg 1984;199:432–7.

[38] Grace PA, Pitt HA, Tompkins RK, et al. Decreased morbidity and mortality after pancreatoduodenectomy. Am J Surg 1986;151:141–9.

[39] Crist DW, Sitzmann JV, Cameron JL. Improved hospital morbidity, mortality, and survival after the Whipple procedure. Ann Surg 1987;206:358–65.

[40] Trede M, Schwall G, Saeger HD. Survival after pancreatoduodenectomy: 118 consecutive resections without an operative mortality. Ann Surg 1990;211:447–58.

[41] Geer RJ, Brennan MF. Prognostic indicators for survival after resection of pancreatic adenocarcinoma. Am J Surg 1993;165:68–72.

[42] Nitecki SS, Sarr MG, Colby TV, et al. Long-term survival after resection for ductal adenocarcinoma of the pancreas: is it really improving? Ann Surg 1995;221:59–66.

[43] Tsao JI, Rossi RL, Lowell JA. Pylorus-preserving pancreatoduodenectomy: is it an adequate cancer operation? Arch Surg 1994;129:405–12.

[44] Yeo CJ, Cameron JL, Maher MM, et al. A prospective randomized trial of pancreaticogastrostomy versus pancreaticojejunostomy after pancreaticoduodenectomy. Ann Surg 1995;222:580–8.

[45] Fernandez-del Castillo C, Rattner DW, et al. Standards for pancreatic resection in the 1990s. Arch Surg 1995;130:295–9.

[46] Yeo CJ, Cameron JL, Sohn TA, et al. Six hundred fifty consecutive pancreaticoduodenectomies in the 1990s: pathology, complications, and outcomes. Ann Surg 1997;226:248–57.

[47] Cameron JL, Pitt HA, Yeo CJ, et al. One hundred and forty-five consecutive pancreaticoduodenectomies without mortality. Ann Surg 1993;217:430–5.

[48] Howard JM. Development and progress in resective surgery for pancreatic cancer. World J Surg 1999;23:901–6.

[49] Cattell RB, Pyrtek LJ. An appraisal of pancreatoduodenal resection: a follow-up study of 61 cases. Ann Surg 1949;129:840–9.

[50] Collins JJ Jr, Craighead JE, Brooks JR. Rationale for total pancreatectomy for carcinoma of the pancreatic head. N Engl J Med 1966;274:599–602.

[51] Rockey EW. Total pancreatectomy for carcinoma: a case report. Ann Surg 1943;118:603–9.
[52] Ross DE. Cancer of the pancreas: a plea for total pancreatectomy. Am J Surg 1954;87: 820–9.
[53] Howard JM, Jordan GL, Reber HA, editors. Surgical disease of the pancreas. Philadelphia: Lea & Febiger; 1978.
[54] Pliam MB, ReMine WH. Further evaluation of total pancreatectomy. Arch Surg 1975;110: 506–12.
[55] Ihse I, Lilja P, Arnesjo B, et al. Total pancreatectomy for cancer: an appraisal of 65 cases. Ann Surg 1977;186:675–80.
[56] Brooks JR, Brooks DC, Levine JD. Total pancreatectomy for ductal cell carcinoma of the pancreas: an update. Ann Surg 1989;209:405–10.
[57] McDermott WV Jr. A one-stage pancreatoduodenectomy with resection of the portal vein for carcinoma of the pancreas. Ann Surg 1952;136:1012–8.
[58] Fortner JG. Regional resection of cancer of the pancreas: a new surgical approach. Surgery 1973;73:307–20.
[59] Fortner JG, Kim DK, Cubilla A, et al. Regional pancreatectomy: en bloc pancreatic, portal vein and lymph node resection. Ann Surg 1977;186:42–50.
[60] Sindelar WF. Clinical experience with regional pancreatectomy for adenocarcinoma of the pancreas. Arch Surg 1989;124:127–32.
[61] Fortner JG, Klimstra DS, Senie RT, et al. Tumor size is the primary prognosticator for pancreatic cancer after regional pancreatectomy. Ann Surg 1996;223:147–53.
[62] Nagakawa T, Konishi I, Ueno K, et al. Surgical treatment of pancreatic cancer: the Japanese experience. International Journal of Pancreatology: official journal of IAP 1991;9: 135–43.
[63] Harrison LE, Klimstra DS, Brennan MF. Isolated portal vein involvement in pancreatic adenocarcinoma: a contraindication for resection? Ann Surg 1996;224:342–7.
[64] Leach SD, Lee JE, Charnsangavej C, et al. Survival following pancreaticoduodenectomy with resection of the superior mesenteric-portal vein confluence for adenocarcinoma of the pancreatic head. Br J Surg 1998;85:611–7.
[65] Bold RJ, Charnsangavej C, Cleary KR, et al. Major vascular resection as part of pancreaticoduodenectomy for cancer: Radiologic, intraoperative, and pathologic analysis. J Gastrointest Surg 1999;3:233–43.
[66] Nagakawa T, Mori K, Nakano T, et al. Perineural invasion of carcinoma of the pancreas and biliary tract. Br J Surg 1993;80:619–21.
[67] Fuhrman GM, Leach SD, Staley CA, et al, for the Pancreatic Tumor Study Group. Rationale for en bloc vein resection in the treatment of pancreatic adenocarcinoma adherent to the superior mesenteric-portal vein confluence. Ann Surg 1996;223:154–62.
[68] The Gastrointestinal Tumor Study Group. A multi-institutional comparative trial of radiation therapy alone and in combination with 5-fluorouracil for locally unresectable pancreatic carcinoma. Ann Surg 1979;189:205–8.
[69] Pisters PW, Evans DB, Leung DH, et al. Surgery for ductal adenocarcinoma of the pancreatic head. World J Surg 2001;25:533–4.
[70] Rosch T, Dittler HJ, Strobel K, et al. Endoscopic ultrasound criteria for vascular invasion in the staging of cancer of the head of the pancreas: a blind reevaluation of videotapes. Gastrointest Endosc 2000;52:469–77.
[71] Ishikawa O, Ohhigashi H, Sasaki Y, et al. Practical usefulness of lymphatic and connective tissue clearance for the carcinoma of the pancreas head. Ann Surg 1988;208:215–20.
[72] Manabe T, Ohshio G, Baba N, et al. Radical pancreatectomy for ductal cell carcinoma of the head of the pancreas. Cancer 1989;64:1132–7.
[73] Pedrazzoli S, DiCarlo V, Dionigi R, et al, for the Lymphadenectomy Study Group. Standard versus extended lymphadenectomy associated with pancreatoduodenectomy in the surgical treatment of adenocarcinoma of the head of the pancreas: a multicenter, prospective, randomized study. Ann Surg 1998;228:508–17.

[74] Yeo CJ, Cameron JL, Lillemoe KD, et al. Pancreaticoduodenectomy with or without distal gastrectomy and extended retroperitoneal lymphadenectomy for periampullary adenocarcinoma, part 2: randomized controlled trial evaluating survival, morbidity, and mortality. Ann Surg 2002;236:355–66.

[75] Nguyen TC, Sohn TA, Cameron JL, et al. Standard vs. radical pancreaticoduodenectomy for periampullary adenocarcinoma: a prospective, randomized trial evaluating quality of life in pancreaticoduodenectomy survivors. J Gastrointest Surg 2003;7:1–9.

[76] Traverso LW, Longmire WP Jr. Preservation of the pylorus in pancreaticoduodenectomy. J Am Coll Surg (Surg Gynecol Obstet) 1978;146:959–62.

[77] Di Carlo V, Zerbi A, Balzano G, et al. Pylorus-preserving pancreaticoduodenectomy versus conventional Whipple operation. World J Surg 1999;23:920–5.

[78] Grace PA, Pitt HA, Longmire WP. Pylorus preserving pancreatoduodenectomy: an overview. Br J Surg 1990;77:968–74.

[79] Patel AG, Toyama MT, Kusske AM, et al. Pylorus-preserving Whipple resection for pancreatic cancer: is it any better? Arch Surg 1995;130:838–42.

[80] Klinkenbijl JH, van der Schelling GP, Hop WC, et al. The advantages of pylorus-preserving pancreatoduodenectomy in malignant disease of the pancreas and periampullary region. Ann Surg 1992;216:142–5.

[81] Roder JD, Stein HJ, Huttl W, et al. Pylorus-preserving versus standard pancreaticoduodenectomy: an analysis of 110 pancreatic and periampullary carcinomas. Br J Surg 1992;79:152–5.

[82] Warshaw AL, Torchiana DL. Delayed gastric emptying after pylorus-preserving pancreaticoduodenectomy. J Am Coll Surg 1985;160:1–4.

[83] Hunt DR, McLean R. Pylorus-preserving pancreatectomy: functional results. Br J Surg 1989;76:173–6.

[84] Williamson RC, Bliouras N, Cooper MJ, et al. Gastric emptying and enterogastric reflux after conservative and conventional pancreatoduodenectomy. Surgery 1993;114:82–6.

[85] Yeo CJ, Barry MK, Sauter PK, et al. Erythromycin accelerates gastric emptying after pancreaticoduodenectomy: a prospective, randomized, placebo-controlled trial. Ann Surg 1993;218:229–37.

[86] Kozuschek W, Reith HB, Waleczek H, et al. A comparison of long term results of the standard Whipple procedure and the pylorus preserving pancreatoduodenectomy. J Am Coll Surg 1994;178:443–53.

[87] Lin PW, Lin YJ. Prospective randomized comparison between pylorus-preserving and standard pancreaticoduodenectomy. Br J Surg 1999;86:603–7.

[88] Seiler CA, Wagner M, Sadowski C, et al. Randomized prospective trial of pylorus-preserving vs. classic duodenopancreatectomy (Whipple procedure): initial clinical results. J Gastrointest Surg 2000;4:443–52.

[89] Tran KT, Smeenk HG, van Eijck CH, et al. Pylorus preserving pancreaticoduodenectomy versus standard Whipple procedure: a prospective, randomized, multicenter analysis of 170 patients with pancreatic and periampullary tumors. Ann Surg 2004;240: 738–45.

[90] Chou FF, Sheen-Chen SM, Chen YS, et al. Postoperative morbidity and mortality of pancreaticoduodenectomy for periampullary cancer. Eur J Surg 1996;162:477–81.

[91] Bassi C, Falconi M, Molinari E, et al. Duct-to-mucosa versus end-to-side pancreaticojejunostomy reconstruction after pancreaticoduodenectomy: results of a prospective randomized trial. Surgery 2003;134:766–71.

[92] Yeo CJ, Sohn TA, Cameron JL, et al. Periampullary adenocarcinoma: analysis of 5-year survivors. Ann Surg 1998;227:821–31.

[93] Gudjonsson B. Cancer of the pancreas: 50 years of surgery. Cancer 1987;60:2284–303.

[94] Lieberman MD, Kilburn H, Lindsey M, et al. Relation of perioperative deaths to hospital volume among patients undergoing pancreatic resection for malignancy. Ann Surg 1995; 222:638–45.

[95]   Gordon TA, Burleyson GP, Tielsch JM, et al. The effects of regionalization on cost and
       outcome for one general high-risk surgical procedure. Ann Surg 1995;221:43–9.
[96]   Glasgow RE, Mulvihill SJ. Hospital volume influences outcome in patients undergoing
       pancreatic resection for cancer. Western Journal of Medecine 1996;165:294–300.
[97]   Sosa JA, Bowman HM, Gordon TA, et al. Importance of hospital volume in the overall
       management of pancreatic cancer. Ann Surg 1998;228:429–38.
[98]   Birkmeyer JD, Finlayson SR, Tosteson AN, et al. Effect of hospital volume on in-hospital
       mortality with pancreaticoduodenectomy. Surgery 1999;125:250–6.
[99]   Begg CB, Cramer LD, Hoskins WJ, et al. Impact of hospital volume on operative mortality
       for major cancer surgery. JAMA 1998;280:1747–51.
[100] Simunovic M, To T, Theriault M, et al. Relation between hospital surgical volume and
       outcome for pancreatic resection for neoplasm in a publicly funded health care system.
       CMAJ 1999;160:643–8.
[101] Kingsnorth AN. Major HPB procedures must be undertaken in high volume quaternary
       centres? HPB Surg 2000;11:359–61.
[102] Birkmeyer JD, Siewers AE, Finlayson EV, et al. Hospital volume and surgical mortality in
       the United States. N Engl J Med 2002;346:1128–37.
[103] Ho V, Heslin MJ. Effect of hospital volume and experience on in-hospital mortality for
       pancreaticoduodenectomy. Ann Surg 2003;237:509–14.
[104] Urbach DR, Baxter NN. Does it matter what a hospital is "high volume" for? specificity of
       hospital volume-outcome associations for surgical procedures: analysis of administrative
       data. BMJ 2004;328:737–40.
[105] Birkmeyer JD, Stukel TA, Siewers AE, et al. Surgeon volume and operative mortality in the
       United States. N Engl J Med 2003;349:2117–27.
[106] Swartz MJ, Batra SK, Varshney GC, et al. MUC4 expression increases progressively in
       pancreatic intraepithelial neoplasia. Am J Clin Pathol 2002;117:791–6.

ELSEVIER
SAUNDERS

Surg Oncol Clin N Am
14 (2005) 553–568

SURGICAL
ONCOLOGY CLINICS
OF NORTH AMERICA

Evolution of Radical Procedures for Urologic Cancer

Jenne E. Garrett, MD[a],
Randall G. Rowland, MD, PhD[b],*

[a]Division of Urology, University of Kentucky Chandler Medical Center,
800 Rose Street, MS 277, Lexington, KY 40536-0298, USA
[b]Division of Urology, University of Kentucky Chandler Medical Center,
800 Rose Street, MS 283, Lexington, KY 40536-0298, USA

Kidney

Renal cell carcinoma represents 2% of adult cancers and is the third most common genitourinary malignancy. Its classic presentation of flank pain, flank mass, and hematuria occurs in approximately 10% of the cases. Jayson and Sanders [1] found only 1 of 131 patients presented with the classic triad. With the advent of new imaging modalities, particularly CT and MRI, the number of renal masses discovered incidentally has increased to the point that they now represent the majority [1,2].

What is described today as a simple nephrectomy was the procedure performed for renal cell carcinoma up until 1948 when Mortensen [3] described a radical nephrectomy, defined as the removal of all contents within Gerota's, fascia including the kidney, adrenal glands, and perirenal fat. In 1963, Robson [4] advocated performing a regional lymphadenectomy with the radical nephrectomy after observing that 22.5% of 62 nephrectomies for renal cell carcinoma showed involvement of the lymphatics surrounding the renal hilum. In 1969, Robson published convincing results demonstrating a significant survival advantage in 88 patients regardless of tumor size when regional lymphadenectomy was combined with radical nephrectomy [5]. This new definition of radical nephrectomy with regional lymphadenectomy has remained relatively unchanged since that time, except for the preservation of the ipsilateral adrenal gland in selected cases. Because renal cell carcinoma is radio- and chemotherapy-resistant, surgical

---

* Corresponding author.
E-mail address: rrowlan@uky.edu (R.G. Rowland).

removal has remained the mainstay of therapy, although several minimally invasive experimental techniques including cryotherapy, high intensity focused ultrasonography, and radiofrequency ablation have recently demonstrated improved cure rates [6].

The first laparoscopic nephrectomy was performed in 1990 by Clayman and colleagues [7]. Initially, the value of this procedure for treating renal cancer was in question. As laparoscopic skills improved, multiple centers began performing this procedure, changing the indications from non-cancerous to cancerous lesions. In 2000, Dunn and colleagues [8] published their 9-year experience comparing the laparoscopic approach with open nephrectomy. They found a statistically significant decrease in blood loss, hospital stay, and pain requirement and a faster return to normal activity in the laparoscopically treated group, although this approach cost more and required more time to perform. There was no difference found in the recurrence of 8% to 9% between the two groups at 2 years' follow-up. Major complications likewise differed by 3.3% in the laparoscopic group versus 12% in the open group, although the average mass size in the open group was 7.4 cm versus 5.3 cm in the laparoscopic group. Likewise, long-term studies have demonstrated that there is no increased risk of port site or renal fossa recurrence or tumor spillage with the laparoscopic approach [6,8–10].

The first partial nephrectomy for renal cell carcinoma was performed by Czerny in 1887. Because of significant postoperative morbidity, this approach was abandoned until recently, with the advances in imaging modalities, infection control, and improved surgical techniques [11]. Originally, open partial nephrectomy was used only for bilateral disease, a mass in a solitary kidney, or renal insufficiency [12]. Now, with more than 10 years of follow-up, partial nephrectomy for renal tumors in anatomically favorable locations less than 4 cm has the same perioperative morbidity rate, cancer control efficacy, and outcomes as radical nephrectomy. The recurrence rate in this tumor size is 0% to 3% and has been found to be the result of multicentricity rather than insufficient resection [11,13,14]. Partial nephrectomies for tumors greater than 4 cm have been shown to have decreased 5- and 10-year survival rates, regardless of the negative margin status at the time of resection [15].

Another advantage associated with partial nephrectomy is the decreased risk of renal insufficiency, regardless of preoperative comorbidities. McKiernan and colleagues [16] followed 173 patients for 25 months and found that those who had undergone radical nephrectomy showed a mean creatinine level of 1.5, whereas those who had undergone partial nephrectomy showed a mean creatinine level of 1.0 [12].

Unfortunately, many of the benefits of laparoscopy, including decreased blood loss, pain, and hospital stay, were lost with the open partial nephrectomy (OPN). To regain the benefits from laparoscopy, teaching institutions have integrated the laparoscopic partial nephrectomy (LPN). Although the procedure is technically challenging, efforts have been made to mimic open surgery, which has produced similar cancer control results.

Bhayani and colleagues [17] have summarized the shift from open radical nephrectomy to laparoscopic nephrectomy to open partial nephrectomy to laparoscopic partial nephrectomy in reviewing 537 patients who underwent surgery for renal malignancy. By 2001, laparoscopic radical nephrectomy was the standard of care for TNM stage T1 and T2 lesions. An analysis of the percentage of partial nephrectomies performed before and after the popularity of laparoscopic radical nephrectomy shows this procedure has remained unchanged at approximately 40%. This consistent percentage, despite the steady increase in the number of laparoscopic nephrectomies performed, demonstrates that kidneys are not be removed laparoscopically that can be managed with nephron-sparing surgery.

With recent advances in laparoscopic instrumentation, tissue sealants, and intracorporeal suturing, laparoscopic partial nephrectomy has become more feasible. Gill and colleagues [18] have compared 100 laparoscopic and 100 open partial nephrectomy cases from the Cleveland Clinic. Larger tumors were more common in the open group, whereas older patients were more common in the laparoscopic group. There was an increase in warm ischemia times, a decrease in operating room times, blood loss, narcotic use, and hospital stay, and patients returned more rapidly to baseline functioning in the LPN group compared with the OPN group. The overall complication rates were the same between the two groups, but there was an increased risk of major complications in the laparoscopic group of 5% versus 0%, including three cases of bleeding and one case of ureteral injury. There were three cases of positive margins in the laparoscopic group compared with none in the open group. No laparoscopic case was converted to open surgery. Although LPN is becoming used more widely, increased care must be taken to ensure negative margins to achieve long-term results similar to OPN.

Several minimally invasive techniques are being evaluated for treating small renal lesions, including cryotherapy, high intensity focused ultrasonography, and radio frequency ablation. These techniques are being evaluated presently for long-term success rates, and they remain experimental and limited to patients with surgically prohibitive comorbid conditions [19].

Currently, laparoscopic radical nephrectomy is the standard of care for T1a–T3a lesions, with equivalent cancer control comparable to open nephrectomy. Nephron-sparing surgery is the standard of care for localized renal cell carcinoma in patients with clinical circumstances that warrant the preservation of renal function and is fast becoming so for small peripheral renal lesions in patients with normal contralateral kidneys. To date, cancer-free survival is the same for nephron-sparing surgery as it is for radical nephrectomy [20]. OPN is still the gold standard for nephron-sparing surgery, although LPN is gaining wider acceptance as instruments and the ability to control bleeding and the positive margin rate are improving. Although laparoscopy has gained dominance in renal surgery, there are still indications for open radical nephrectomy, including inferior vena caval involvement of the tumor, local tumor invasion, massive size, and gross lymphadenopathy. Attempts to perform laparoscopic nephrectomy for the above situations have led to an increased complication rate, conversion to open surgery, and increased operating room times [20].

Adrenal

The first adrenal gland, removed in 1859 by Thornton, was a 20-lb specimen removed en bloc with the kidney. The first planned adrenalectomy was performed in 1914 by Sargent, who removed a 17-cm adenoma from a patient with Cushing's syndrome. The first pheochromocytoma was removed by Charles Mayo, in 1927, through a flank incision. Young, in 1936, was the first to describe bilateral adrenalectomies through a posterior approach for a patient with metastatic prostate cancer and primary hyperaldosteronism [21]. Initially, the major complications were hemorrhage and infection. The transperitoneal, retroperitoneal, and transthoracic approaches have all been described, and indications for each approach depend on the tumor location and size, body habitus, patient comorbidities, and surgeon preference. Surgical resection is advocated for tumors greater than 5 cm, those with heterogeneity, irregular borders, calcifications, regional lymphadenopathy, suspicious fine needle biopsy aspirates, or a lack of microlipids as observed on chemical shift MRI. The size limit cutoff is lowered to 3 cm for healthy younger patients or tumors that increase in size over time. Tumors between 3 and 5 cm with benign features are followed conservatively in elderly or less healthy patients [22].

The first laparoscopic adrenalectomy was reported in 1992 by Gagner and coworkers [23]. As surgical expertise improved, reports comparing open versus laparoscopic adrenalectomy appeared, demonstrating improved complication rates and decreased hospital stay, narcotic requirement, and estimated blood loss. Operative times were slightly higher but decreased as surgical skills improved. Within 10 years of its description, laparoscopic adrenalectomy has become the standard of care for most adrenal gland disease [24–27].

Initially, absolute contraindications to laparoscopic adrenalectomy included pheochromocytomas, malignant adrenal lesions, and tumors greater than 6 to 10 cm. As skills improved and long-term results demonstrated adequate control of functioning adrenal tumors, the indications have widened. Currently, lesion size is not a contraindication, although laparoscopic treatment of adrenal lesions greater than 12 to 13 cm is rare [28]. Invasive adrenocortical carcinoma lesions are still treated in an open fashion because they require en bloc resection of the kidney, perinephric and adrenal fat, lymph nodes, diaphragm, and occasionally the tail of the pancreas. Likewise, malignant pheochromocytomas and symptomatic adrenal masses in pregnant women are still managed in an open fashion. Porpiglia and colleagues [28] studied laparoscopic adrenalectomies performed with pathologic analysis that demonstrated adrenal cortical carcinoma or metastasis and found that at 30-month follow-up, one of 14 patients developed local port site seeding from nonsmall-cell lung cancer metastasis to the adrenal gland, and one patient showed distant thoracic invasion from a breast cancer primary. One of 14 patients required conversion to an open procedure because of periadrenal spread and the need for an en-bloc resection of the kidney and adjacent structures that was not appreciated on preoperative imaging studies. The complication rate, hospital stay, pain, and convalescence were all improved through the laparoscopic approach. The authors concluded that in a patient with adequately controlled primary malignancy and isolated metastasis to the adrenal or primary adrenal cortical carcinoma confined to the adrenal gland, laparoscopic adrenalectomy is feasible.

Laparoscopic adrenalectomy can be performed through various approaches similar to open adrenalectomy. The approach chosen depends on surgical preference, tumor size, location, body habitus, and patient comorbidities. The lateral transperitoneal approach is used frequently because it allows dissected structures to fall away from the adrenal gland. The identification of the adrenal vein is paramount as is dissection of the patient away from the mass, particularly with functional adrenal gland lesions [22,26].

Laparoscopic adrenalectomy has become the standard of care for most adrenal lesions. Appropriate hormonal evaluation before removal is important and helps with preoperative preparation and surgical planning. Absolute contraindications are changing as laparoscopic skills improve. Open surgery is still the gold standard for invasive adrenal cortical carcinoma.

Bladder

Radical cystectomy has been the standard procedure for muscle-invasive bladder cancer since the early 1900s. Survival has dramatically increased in the last several decades, based on improved anesthesia, blood banking, antibiotics, suture materials, and stapling devices. Based on lower mortality and morbidity rates for radical cystectomy and the appreciation of the aggressive behavior of high-grade T1 tumors, the indications for cystectomy have been expanded to this group of patients, especially for those who have failed intravesical therapy [29].

One exception to this trend has been the use of radical or very aggressive transurethral resection of bladder tumors (TUR-BT) in patients with superficial (T1) and even muscle invasion (T2) who are not candidates for an extirpative procedure or who refuse cystectomy. The aggressive TUR-BT procedure also has been used in chemo-radiation therapy protocols for organ preservation [30].

The basic techniques of cystectomy have not changed significantly over the last several decades; however, four areas have undergone or are undergoing change. Recently, the extent of lymphadenectomy has been examined. Some authors have advocated more extensive lymphadenectomies, extending up to the bifurcation of the aorta and even to the periaortic area [31,32]. Quek and colleagues [32] suggest that patients may enjoy an increased survival rate related to the number of lymph nodes removed.

The second area of major evolution has been the types of urinary diversion or urinary reconstruction that are available to the patients. Historically, the first urinary diversion was the ureterosigmoidostomy, described in 1852 by Simon [33]. Very few diversions or reconstructions were performed until the 1920s or 1930s. In 1929, Hammer [34] reported the development of colon cancer in a patient who had undergone a ureterosigmoidostomy. The ileal conduit became the standard type of urinary diversion in the 1950s and 1960s [35]. In the 1970s, a continent cutaneous urinary reservoir was reported by Kock [36].

In the 1970s, Camey and colleagues [37] developed the nondetubularized ileal neobladder. The work of Kock [36] emphasized the importance of detubularizing bowel segments used for a urine storage function to decrease the intrareservoir pressure and to increase the capacity of the reservoir without having to use a lengthy segment of bowel. Over the next two decades, many different techniques of continent cutaneous urinary diversions and neobladder reconstructions have been described. In the past decade, the most frequent continent cutaneous urinary diversions that are used are made from the detubularized right colon (the Indiana [38] and the MAINZ pouch [39]). The most frequent neobladder reconstructions are created by using ileum (the hemi-Kock [40], Struder neobladder, [41] and the Hautmann neobladder [42]).

The third evolving area is the exploration of sparing not only potency but also ejaculatory function. In carefully selected patients, the seminal vesicles and all of the supra-ampullary portion of the prostate have been spared [43,44]. Meinhardt and Horenblas [43] reported potency in 19 of 24 patients without any other treatment. Half of the patients experienced antegrade ejaculation. Terrone and colleagues [44] reported potency in 26 of 28 patients, with antegrade ejaculation in 15 (53.5%) of the patients. The need for stringent patient selection for these procedures cannot be overemphasized.

Currently, descriptions of the adaptation of minimally invasive surgical (MIS) techniques to radical cystectomy and urinary diversion or reconstruction are being published [45,46]. Many procedures involve performing the cystectomy portion laparoscopically and the division portion open. As techniques and instruments improve, MIS techniques will almost certainly become widely used for cystectomies.

Prostate

Prostate cancer is the most commonly diagnosed cancer of men in the United States, with one in six men diagnosed during their lifetime.

Prostate cancer represents one third of all new cancer cases each year. Before the 1980s, over half of men had metastatic disease at the time of diagnosis, whereas in 2004, 83% of men have localized disease at diagnosis. Although 31,000 males die of prostate cancer each year, the death rate has been decreasing by 4% per year since 1994, and there has been a 20% increase in 5-year prostate cancer survival rates from 1985 to 1995 [22,47,48].

The first surgical interventions for prostate cancer were performed to relieve obstruction, dating as far back as 1639. These operations were performed through a perineal approach. Several pioneers studied enucleation of the lateral and median lobes of the prostate through the perineum, with Goodfellow credited as the first to successfully perform perineal prostatectomies on a routine basis [49]. In 1904, Young [50] described a systematic approach to a radical perineal prostatectomy (RPP) for treating prostate cancer, which became the standard approach for over 40 years until the introduction of the radical retropubic prostatectomy (RRP). In 1945, Millin introduced the retropubic approach to radical prostatectomy, with the advantages of access to pelvic lymph nodes. This approach was used initially for benign disease but with modifications was used for cancer control [47]. Because of significant morbidities associated with the retropubic approach, including bleeding, incontinence, and impotency, it did not gain widespread use until the landmark report by Walsh, which describes the anatomic radical prostatectomy in 1983 [51]. In fact, because of substantial complications from radical prostatectomy, external beam radiotherapy gained popularity as a prostate cancer treatment modality because of its limited morbidities until an improvement in surgical approach significantly decreased postoperative complications [52]. Through Walsh's research on fresh and stillborn cadavers, the anatomy of the dorsal venous complex and neurovascular bundles were more thoroughly defined, and techniques for improved control and preservation were described. He followed 1623 men for over 10 years after they had undergone radical prostatectomy and found that the preservation of sexual function did not compromise cancer control, with the overall actuarial cause-specific survival rate of 99% and 93%, respectively, at 5 and 10 years' follow-up. Overall postoperative potency rates were 68%, and postoperative continence rates were 92% [53]. These data have been validated by other series [54,55].

The need to find a better modality for diagnosing prostate cancer, while still confined to the gland, resulted in the purification of prostate-specific antigen (PSA) in 1979, which was subsequently approved by the Food and Drug Administration (FDA) in 1985 as a way to monitor prostate cancer. This blood test along with the advent of transrectal ultrasound-guided prostate biopsy, which gained FDA approval in 1994 for the screening of prostate cancer, led to an increased public and physician awareness, improved diagnostic accuracy, and a shift away from initially diagnosing prostate cancer as metastatic to organ confined [47].

The radical perineal prostatectomy (RPP) has regained popularity in the 1990s with the trend toward minimally invasive surgery. Shorter hospital stay and recovery time, the advent of PSA combined with pathologic biopsy grading to stratify the risk of lymph node involvement, an increased number of patients being diagnosed with organ-confined prostate cancer, and the development of a nerve-sparing approach for the perineal prostatectomy all led to its increased use [56,57]. Weldon and colleagues [57] reported on 220 consecutive radical perineal prostatectomies and demonstrated a 95% continence rate by 10 months and potency rate of 70% at 24 months in those patients who had undergone the bilateral nerve-sparing technique. Median blood loss was 600 mL, with total hospital stay of 2 days.

Many urologists have not received formal training in perineal prostatectomy because of its decreased use after the description of the retropubic technique. Likewise, there are concerns that it is more difficult to learn than the retropubic approach and is associated with a higher risk of rectal injury. Mokulis and Thompson [58] reviewed the surgical logs of six graduating urology residents who performed 10 radical perineal and retropubic prostatectomies. They found that the perineal approach was learned more quickly and had decreased complication rates and shorter hospital stay compared with the retropubic approach.

The first laparoscopic radical prostatectomy (LRP) was performed by Raboy and colleagues, in 1997 [59]. Schuessler and colleagues [60] also published their initial results on transperitoneal laparoscopic radical prostatectomy in 1997. The operative times were significantly longer than the other radical prostatectomy techniques, without any significant improvement in continence, potency, or hospital stay. Subsequent studies comparing RRP, RPP, and LRP did not demonstrate any significant advantages over the laparoscopic approach, with a significant increase in operative times [36,37,61–63]. Salomon and colleagues [61] reviewed 401 patients who had undergone radical prostatectomy by retropubic, perineal, or laparoscopic approach and found that the RRP group had a higher transfusion rate, longer bladder catheterization rate, and longer hospital stay. Complication rates were similar, as were positive margin rates in pT2 tumors of 19%, 14%, and 22% respectively. Three-year survival rates were similar among the three groups of patients with organ-confined disease. Guillonneau and colleagues [64] analyzed 1000 LRP cases that demonstrated a positive surgical margin rate of 6.9%, 18.6%, and 30%, respectively, for pT2a, pT2b, and pT3a prostate cancer. The overall actuarial biochemical progression-free survival rate was 90.5% at 3 years' follow-up. They demonstrated that LRP in skilled hands resulted in adequate local tumor control.

Rassweiler and colleagues [65] compared RRP with LRP and demonstrated that 219 patients in the RRP group experienced higher rates of blood loss, transfusion, complications (lymphoceles, wound infection, and embolism), and anastomotic strictures compared with 438 LRP patients.

Continence and positive margin rates were similar in both groups. Postoperative narcotic use was higher with the RRP group. The operative time decreased significantly in the LRP group after performing the first 219 LRP. These studies indicate that LRP provides adequate cancer control compared with other modalities. It is technically challenging and is associated with longer operative times but decreased blood loss and narcotic usage, along with shorter return to baseline function. Whether this approach will result in better continence and potency rates is still being debated. Randomized studies comparing the three modalities will be difficult to perform because surgeon preference and expertise and patient disease and body habitus are considered before choosing a surgical option for the patient.

Penis

Squamous cell carcinoma is the most common cancer of the penis [66]. This is a rare disease, comprising 0.4% to 0.6% of all malignancies diagnosed among males. Surgical excision of the malignant lesion with a margin of normal tissue was advocated first by Celsus in the first century AD. In 1875, Thiersch gave the first in-depth description of excision therapy to cure localized penile malignancy. Not until the 19th century did research establish the pattern of lymph node spread for malignancies that was applied to penile cancer in 1886 by MacCormack, who advocated total penectomy with bilateral lymphadenectomy to cure penile cancer. The morbidities of these procedures were significant. Later in 1948, Daseler published a description of more exact anatomy of the lymph chains draining the penis, after studying 450 cadavers. In the same year, Buonofsky described transposition of the sartorius muscle to decrease the morbidity of radical lymphadenectomy. Cabanos, in 1977, published data suggesting that obtaining a biopsy of the sentinel node was adequate for determining whether to proceed with lymphadenectomy. This technique has largely fallen out of favor because incidences of subsequent metastatic disease with negative sentinel node biopsy have been reported [67]. In 1988, Catalona [68] published results regarding a modified inguinal lymphadenectomy, which targeted the superior medial quadrant, where the highest percentage of positive nodes is found. This modified approach decreased the length of the incision, allowed deeper skin flaps, preserved the saphenous vein, and did not transpose the sartorius muscle, thus decreasing the morbidity associated with the standard groin dissection. In his initial six patients, the modified technique did not compromise cancer control, although it was stressed that this method should be used only with clinically negative or minimally positive nodes.

Penile cancer, if left untreated, results in death in most patients within 2 to 3 years. Biopsy-proven squamous cell carcinoma is required before determining the best treatment option for the patient. This can be performed at the time of the planned excision or separately. Excisional therapy remains the mainstay of treatment because chemotherapy and radiation therapy have limited response rates [51,69,70]. Distal preputial cancer can be treated with wide circumcision, leaving 2-cm margins free of tumor, but this procedure is associated with high recurrence rates, necessitating close follow-up [71,72]. Mohs micrographic surgery also has been used for glans and shaft lesions to achieve negative margins with preservation of skin, but this procedure usually is restricted to more superficial lesions [73,74]. For invasive lesions of the glans and distal shaft, partial penectomy with a 1.5- to 2.0-cm margin free of tumor is the treatment of choice, which has a recurrence rate of 0% to 6% [71]. For more proximal lesions, a total penectomy with perineal urethrostomy is the standard. Thus, stage I cancers that are not poorly differentiated can be treated with partial penectomy, with close follow-up without groin node dissection.

Penile cancer spreads to groin lymph nodes and is relatively unique because the removal of involved groin lymph nodes, if confined, is curative [70]. The foreskin and shaft skin drain to the superficial inguinal region. The glans and corpora drain to the deep inguinal and iliac lymph nodes. The role and timing of inguinal lymphadenectomy has generated significant controversy because the clinical staging of groin lymphadenopathy in patients with penile cancer is notoriously unreliable, and groin dissection is associated with significant morbidity. Twenty percent of palpably negative groin nodes are positive on removal, whereas 50% of palpably positive nodes are negative at removal [54]. Because of the significant morbidity of the radical groin dissection, including lymphedema, hemorrhage, skin flap necrosis, phlebitis, pulmonary embolus, and deep venous thrombosis, many surgeons have advocated delaying node dissection until nodes are palpable. McDougal and colleagues [70] followed 65 patients with penile cancer for 5 years and found an 88% 5-year survival rate for patients with T2 cancers that were treated initially with lymphadenectomy compared with a 38% survival rate for those treated in a delayed fashion. Sixteen percent of patients showed significant lymphedema, and 12% required a second procedure for wound closure. Based on these data, performing lymphade-nectomy on patients with T2 and T3 disease was recommended regardless of lymph node status. These data, which support immediate rather than delayed lymphadenectomy, were validated by Fraley and colleagues [75] in their evaluation of 58 patients.

If the groin nodes are positive, iliac node dissection also should be preformed. It is rare to have positive pelvic nodes without positive inguinal nodes, but histologically positive deep inguinal nodes are associated with 30% positive pelvic nodes. Because of the anatomical crossover of lymphatics, 50% of clinically negative contralateral groins have metastatic disease, thus necessitating bilateral dissection [67].

The modified inguinal lymph node dissection described by Catalona and colleagues [68] has gained popularity in treating clinically negative T2 disease or minimally palpable positive nodes because of its decreased morbidity. D'Ancona and colleagues [76] compared modified with radical lymph node dissection in 26 patients and found a complication rate of 87.5% and 38.9%, respectively. Also, performing lymph node dissection at the time of penectomy was not associated with a higher complication rate. The authors did observe two (7.7%) recurrences in 2 years, which were believed to be caused by positive nodes outside the field of modified dissection.

Nelson and colleagues [77] evaluated 22 patients. They proposed an early ambulation protocol after lymphadenectomy to reduce the risk of deep venous thrombosis and pulmonary embolus. Patients were on bed rest for 8 hours and ambulating after 1 day. All patients wore sequential compression devices and elastic stockings. The study results included a 40% early minor complication rate (less than 30 days after surgery) and a 5% late minor complication rate; no major early complications; but had a 5% late major complication rate (one instance of flap necrosis and one lymphocele that required percutaneous drainage). Because of their results at Vanderbilt University, the authors recommend lymphadenectomy for T2 or greater penile cancer, regardless of palpable lymph nodes. T1 patients undergo lymphadenectomy if they have palpable nodes after 6 weeks of antibiotics. Pelvic lymphadenectomy is restricted to those patients with positive CT scan findings or grossly positive nodes on ilioinguinal lymphadenectomy.

With its reduced morbidity without compromise to cancer control, modified lymphadenectomy has gained popularity. Likewise, because data have demonstrated impressive differences in survival in patients with immediate versus delayed lymphadenectomy for T2 disease, this procedure has become the standard. There does not seem to be a significant risk to performing this simultaneously with partial or total penectomy.

Testis

Surgery for testicular cancer has evolved significantly over the last 4 decades. The necessity of performing a radical orchiectomy through an inguinal approach to allow removal of the spermatic cord structures to the level of the internal inguinal ring without causing any potential cross contamination with the superficial inguinal lymphatics has been appreciated for virtually this entire period. The general pattern of lymphatic drainage of the testicles has been known since the 1910s [78]; however, the extent of the margins of retroperitoneal lymph node dissection (RPLND) remained limited [79] until the 1960s and 1970s when the extent of dissection was increased based on the clinical observations of Donohue [80].

The development of an effective systemic *cis*-diamminedichloroplatinum (cisplatin)–based chemotherapy dramatically improved survival rates in patients with advanced or bulky metastatic testicular cancer. The role of surgery was redefined in this era of effective chemotherapy. RPLND was used as a staging and therapeutic procedure in low-stage disease and as an adjuvant or salvage procedure in patients with bulky or disseminated disease who did not achieve a complete response with chemotherapy.

During the peak of its usage, the RPLND borders of dissection were defined as the diaphragm cranially, the ureters laterally, and the bifurcation of the common iliac arteries caudally [80]. Although this procedure could be performed with a low mortality rate ($\leq 1\%$) and low morbidity and reoperation rates in patients undergoing the procedure for low-stage disease, virtually all patients were rendered infertile at the time based on the loss of emission of seminal fluid secondary to the sympathectomy, which resulted from the extensive bilateral fields of dissection.

In the mid to late 1980s, several centers began looking at modifying the templates and developing a prospective nerve-sparing techniques to save the lumbar sympathetic chains and post-ganglionic branches to preserve normal seminal emission and, thus, antegrade ejaculation [81–83].

A consensus exists that the margins for dissection for clinically low-stage testicular cancer is the renal vessels cranially, the ipsilateral ureter and the midsagittal plane of the contralateral great vessel laterally, and the ipsilateral common iliac artery caudally. The area around the origin of the inferior mesenteric artery is spared for both a right- and left-sided dissection.

These modified templates allow the preservation of the entire contralateral sympathetic chain and post-ganglionic branches. The use of a prospective "split and roll" nerve-sparing technique within the field of dissection allows preservation of the ipsilateral sympathetics. The use of the modified template of dissection and the prospective nerve-sparing techniques allows the preservation of emission of antegrade ejaculation in 98% to 100% of the patients [84].

In the setting of a post-chemotherapy RPLND, a full bilateral template dissection is recommended. However, it is possible that the contralateral side may be able to be dissected using a nerve-sparing technique if there has never been any gross disease within that area during the course of the patient's treatment. In that case 76.5% of the patients will have preservation of emission with antegrade ejaculation [85].

RPLND will render up to 60% of patients with low-stage, low-volume metastatic testicular cancer free of disease, without any other additional treatment. RPLND in the post-chemotherapy setting will make many of the patients with cancer that remains after primary chemotherapy disease free. Those patients who have teratoma remaining after chemotherapy also benefit from RPLND when complete excision of residual masses can be accomplished.

As in most of the other organs in urology, MIS is affecting the treatment of testicular cancer. Laparoscopic techniques have been used in centers of advanced MIS for more than 10 years [86]. One hundred twenty procedures were performed as the primary treatment, and 68 procedures were performed in the post-chemotherapy setting. Emission and antegrade ejaculation were present in 98.4% of patients. Only six of the 120 patients with low-stage disease were found to be relapsed at greater than 4 years' follow-up. A small series experience of laparoscopic RPLND in the post-chemotherapy setting also has been reported by Hara and associates [87].

The role of RPLND in the treatment of testicular cancer in the future will be determined by balancing the morbidity, mortality, cost, and recurrence rates after surgery with the morbidity, mortality, effect on fertility, recurrence rates, and rates of the development of secondary tumors or other chronic illness after exposure to chemotherapy. The development of better markers and predictors of biologic potential of these tumors also will play a role in determining the type and extent of treatment used for testicular cancer.

References

[1] Jayson M, Sanders H. Increased incidence of serendipitously discovered renal cell carcinoma. Urology 1998;51:204–5.
[2] Skinner DG, Colvin RB, Vermillion CD, et al. Diagnosis and management of renal cell carcinoma: a clinical and pathologic study of 309 cases. Cancer 1971;28:1165–77.
[3] Mortensen H. Transthoracic nephrectomy. J Urol 1948;60:855–8.
[4] Robson CJ. Radical nephrectomy for renal cell carcinoma. J Urol 1963;89:37–42.
[5] Robson CJ, Churchill BM, Anderson W. The results of radical nephrectomy for renal cell carcinoma. J Urol 1969;101:297–301.
[6] Chan DY, Cadeddu JA, Jarrett TW, et al. Laparoscopic radical nephrectomy: cancer control for renal cell carcinoma. J Urol 2001;166:2095–100.
[7] Clayman RV, Kavoussi LR, Soper NJ, et al. Laparoscopic nephrectomy: initial case report. J Urol 1991;146:278–82.
[8] Dunn MD, Portis AJ, Shalhav AL, et al. Laparoscopic versus open radical nephrectomy: a 9-year experience. J Urol 2000;164:1153–9.
[9] Cadeddu JA, Ono Y, Clayman RV, et al. Laparoscopic nephrectomy for renal cell cancer: evaluation of efficacy and safety: a multicenter experience. Urology 1998;52:773–7.
[10] Ono Y, Kinukawa T, Hattori R, et al. Laparoscopic radical nephrectomy for renal cell carcinoma: a five-year experience. Urology 1999;53:280–6.
[11] Uzzo RG, Novick AC. Nephron sparing surgery for renal tumors: indications, techniques and outcomes. J Urol 2001;166:6–18.
[12] Matin SR, Gill IS, Worley S, Novick AC. Outcome of laparoscopic radical and open partial nephrectomy for the sporadic 4 cm or less renal tumor with a normal contralateral kidney. J Urol 2002;168:1356–60.
[13] Lee CT, Katz J, Shi W, et al. Surgical management of renal tumors 4 cm or less in a contemporary cohort. J Urol 2002;163:730–6.
[14] Herr HW. Partial nephrectomy for unilateral renal carcinoma and a normal contralateral kidney: 10-year followup. J Urol 1999;161:33–5.
[15] Hafez KS, Fergany AF, Novick AC. Nephron sparing surgery for localized renal cell carcinoma: impact of tumor size on patient survival, tumor recurrence and TNM staging. J Urol 1999;162:1930–3.
[16] McKiernan J, Simmons R, Katz J, et al. Natural history of chronic renal insufficiency after partial and radical nephrectomy. Urology 2002;59:816–20.
[17] Bhayani SB, Clayman RV, Sundaram CP, et al. Surgical treatment of renal neoplasia: evolving toward a laparoscopic standard of care. Urology 2003;62:821–6.

[18] Gill IS, Matin SF, Desai MM, et al. Comparative analysis of laparoscopic versus open partial nephrectomy for renal tumors in 200 patients. J Urol 2003;170:64–8.

[19] Hines-Peralta A, Goldberg SN. Review of radiofrequency ablation for renal cell carcinoma. Clin Cancer Res 2004;10:6328–34.

[20] Novick AC. Laparoscopic and partial nephrectomy. Clin Cancer Res 2004;10:6322–7.

[21] Guz BV, Straffon RA, Novick AC. Operative approaches to the adrenal gland. Urol Clin North Am 1989;16(3):527–33.

[22] Vaughan ED, Blumenfeld JD, Pizzo JD, et al. The adrenals. In: Walsh PC, Retik AB, Vaughan ED, et al, editors. Campbell's urology. 8th edition. Philadelphia: WB Saunders; 2002. p. 3507–69.

[23] Gagner M, Lacrois A, Bolt E. Laparoscopic adrenalectomy in Cushing's syndrome and pheochromocytoma. NEJM 1992;327:1003–6.

[24] Guazzoni G, Cestari A, Montorsi F, et al. Laparoscopic treatment of adrenal disease: 10 years on. BJU Int 2004;93:221–7.

[25] Gagner M, Pomp A, Todd HB, et al. Laparoscopic adrenalectomy: lessons learned from 100 consecutive procedures. Ann Surg 1997;226(3):238–47.

[26] Gill IS. The case for laparoscopic adrenalectomy. J Urol 2001;166:429–36.

[27] Hallfeldt KJ, Mussack T, Trupka A, et al. Laparoscopic lateral adrenalectomy versus open posterior adrenalectomy for the treatment of benign adrenal tumors. Surg Endosc 2003;17:264–7.

[28] Porpiglia F, Fiori C, Tarabuzzi R, et al. Is laparoscopic adrenalectomy feasible for adrenocortical carcinoma or metatasis? BJU Int 4:94:1026–9.

[29] Hara I, Miyake H, Takechi Y, et al for the Urogenital Tumor Study Group. Clinical outcome of conservative therapy for stage T1, grade 3 transitional cell carcinoma of the bladder. Int J Urol 2003;10(1):19–24.

[30] Grob BM, Macchia RJ. Radical transurethral resection in the management of muscle-invasive bladder cancer. J Endourol 2001;15(4):419–23 [discussion: 425–6].

[31] Sanderson KM, Stein JP, Skinner DG. The evolving role of pelvic lymphadenectomy in the treatment of bladder cancer. Urol Oncol 2004;22(3):205–11 [discussion: 212–3].

[32] Quek ML, Sanderson KM, Daneshmand S, et al. The importance of an extended lymphadenectomy in the management of high-grade invasive bladder cancer. Expert Rev Anticancer Ther 2004;4(6):1007–16.

[33] Simon J. Ectopia vesicae: operation for directing the orifices of the ureters into the rectum. Lancet 1852;2:568.

[34] Hammer E. Cancer du colon sigmoide dix ans après implantation des uretères d'une vessie exstrophique. J Urol Nephrol (Paris) 1929;28:260.

[35] Bricker EM. Bladder substitution after pelvic evisceration. Surg Clin North Am 1950;30:1511.

[36] Kock NG. Ileostomy without external appliances: a survey of 25 provided with intra-abdominal intestinal reservoir. Ann Surg 1971;173:545.

[37] Camey M, Richard F, Botto H. Bladder replacement by ileocystoplasty. In: King LR, Stone AR, Webster GD, editors. Bladder reconstruction and continent urinary diversion. Chicago: Year Book Medical Publishers; 1987. p. 336–59.

[38] Rowland RG, Mitchell ME, Bihrle R, et al. The Indiana continent urinary reservoir. J Urol 1987;137:1136–9.

[39] Thuroff J, Alken P, Riedmiller H, et al. The MAINZ pouch (mixed augmentation ileum and cecum) for bladder augmentation and continent diversion. J Urol 1986;136:17–26.

[40] Skinner DG, Boyd SD, Lieskovsky G, et al. Lower urinary tract reconstruction following cystectomy: experience and results in 126 patients using the Kock ileal reservoir with bilateral ureteroileal urethrostomy. J Urol 1991;146:756–60.

[41] Studer UE, Ackerman D, Casanova GA, et al. Three years' experience with an ideal low pressure bladder substitute. Br J Urol 1989;63:43.

[42] Hautmann RE, Egghart G, Frohneberg D, et al. The ileal neobladder. J Urol 1988;139: 39–42.

[43] Meinhardt W, Horenblas S. Sexuality preserving cystectomy and neobladder (SPCN): functional results of a neobladder anastomosed to the prostate. Eur Urol 2003;43(6): 646–50.

[44] Terrone C, Cracco C, Scarpa RM, et al. Supra-ampullar cystectomy with preservation of sexual function and ileal orthotopic reservoir for bladder tumor: twenty years of experience. Eur Urol 2004;46(2):264–9 [discussion: 269–70].

[45] Gill IS, Kaouk JH, Meraney AM, et al. Laparoscopic radical cystectomy and continent orthotopic ileal neobladder performed completely intraacorporeally: the initial experience. J Urol 2002;168(1):13–8.

[46] Basillote JB, Abdelshehid C, Ahlering TE, et al. Laparoscopic assisted radical cystectomy with ileal neobladder: a comparison with the open approach. J Urol 2004;172(2):489–93.

[47] Denmeade SR, Isaacs JT. Development of prostate cancer treatment: the good news. Prostate 2004;58:211–24.

[48] Jemal A, Murray T, Samuels A, et al. Cancer statistics 2003. CA Cancer J Clin 2003;53:5–26.

[49] Stutzman RE. Open prostatectomy. In: Graham SD Jr, Glenn JF, editors. Glenn's urologic surgery. Philadelphia: Lippincott-Raven; 1998. p. 261–74.

[50] Young JJ. Four cases of radical prostatectomy. Johns Hopkins Bull 1905;16:315.

[51] Walsh PC, Lepor H, Eggleston JC. Radical prostatectomy with preservation of sexual function: anatomical and pathological considerations. Prostate 1983;4:473–85.

[52] Walsh PC. Anatomical radical prostatectomy: evolution of the surgical technique. J Urol 1998;160:2418–24.

[53] Walsh PC, Partin AW, Epstein JI. Cancer control and quality of life following anatomical radical retropubic prostatectomy: results at 10 years. J Urol 1994;152:1831–6.

[54] Maffezzini M, Sevesco M, Taverna G, et al. Evaluation of complications and results in contemporary serious of 300 consecutive radical retropubic prostatectomies with the anatomic approach at a single institution. Urology 2003;61:982–6.

[55] Catalona WJ, Carvalhal GF, Mager DE, et al. Continence and complication rates in 1.870 consecutive radical retropubic prostatectomies. J Urol 1999;162:433–8.

[56] Graham SD. Radical perineal prostatectomy. In: Graham SD Jr, Glenn JF, editors. Glenn's urologic surgery. Philadelphia: Lippincott-Raven; 1998. p. 285–94.

[57] Weldon VE, Tavel FR, Neuwirth H. Continence. potency and morbidity after radical perineal prostatectomy. J Urol 1997;158(4):1470–5.

[58] Mokulis J, Thompson I. Radical prostatectomy: is the perineal approach more difficult to learn? J Urol 1997;157(1):230–2.

[59] Raboy A, Ferzli G, Albert P. Initial experience with extraperitoneal endoscopic radical prostatectomy. Urology 1997;50:849–53.

[60] Schuessler WW, Schulam PG, Clayman RV, et al. Laparoscopic radical prostatectomy: initial short-term experience. Urology 1997;50:854–7.

[61] Salomon L, Levrel O, de la Taille A, et al. Radical prostatectomy by the retropubic perineal and laparoscopic approach: 12 years of experience in one center. Eur Urol 2002;42:103–11.

[62] Salomon L, Levrel O, Anastasiadis AG, et al. Outcome and complications of radical prostatectomy in patients with PSA ≤10 ng/ml: comparison between the retropubic, perineal and laparoscopic approach. Prostate Cancer Prostatic Dis 2002;5:285–90.

[63] Artibani W, Grosso G, Novara G, et al. Is laparoscopic radical prostatectomy better than traditional retropubic radical prostatectomy? an analysis of peri-operative morbidity in two contemporary series in Italy. Eur Urol 2003;44:401–6.

[64] Guillonneau B, El-Fettough H, Baumert H, et al. Laparoscopic radical prostatectomy: oncological evaluation after 1,000 cases at Montsouris Institute. J Urol 2003;169:1261–6.

[65] Rassweiler J, Seemann O, Schulze M, et al. Laparoscopic versus open radical prostatectomy: a comparative study at a single institution. J Urol 2003;169:1689–93.

[66] Rippentrop JM, Joslyn SA, Konety BR. Squamous cell carcinoma of the penis. Cancer 2004;
     101(6):1357–63.
[67] Crawford ED, Daneshgari F. Management of regional lymphatic drainage in carcinoma of
     the penis. Urol Clin North Am 1992;19(2):305–17.
[68] Catalona WJ. Modified inguinal lymphadenectomy for carcinoma of the penis with
     preservation of saphenous veins: technique and preliminary results. J Urol 1988;140:306–9.
[69] Freeman JA, Mohler JL. Inguinal lymphadenectomy for penile carcinoma. In: Glen's
     urologic surgery. Philadelphia: Lippincott-Raven; 1998. p. 559–64.
[70] McDougal WS, Kirchner FK, Edwards RH, et al. Treatment of carcinoma of the penis: the
     case for primary lymphadenectomy. J Urol 1986;136:38–41.
[71] Das S. Penile amputations for the management of primary carcinoma of the penis. Urol Clin
     North Am 1992;19(2):277–98.
[72] Hardner GJ, Bhanalaph T, Murphy GP, et al. Carcinoma of the penis: analysis of therapy in
     100 consecutive cases. J Urol 1972;108:428.
[73] Mohs FE, Snow SN, Larson PO. Mohs micrographic surgery for penile tumors. Urol Clin
     North Am 1992;19:291–304.
[74] Mohs FE, Snow SN, Messing EM, et al. Microscopically controlled surgery in the treatment
     of carcinoma of the penis. J Urol 1985;133:961–6.
[75] Fraley EE, Zhang G, Manivel C, et al. The role of ilioinguinal lymphadenectomy and
     significance of histological differentiation in treatment of carcinoma of the penis. J Urol
     1989;142:1478–82.
[76] D'Ancona CA, Goncalves de Lucena R, Agusto de Oliveria Querne F, et al. Long-term
     followup of penile carcinoma treated with penectomy and bilateral modified inguinal
     lymphadenectomy. J Urol 2004;172:498–501.
[77] Nelson BA, Cookson MS, Smith JA, et al. Complications of inguinal and pelvic
     lymphadenectomy for squamous cell carcinoma of the penis: a contemporary series.
     J Urol 2004;172:494–7.
[78] Jamiesen JK, Dobson JF. The lymphatics of the testicle. Lancet 1910;1:493.
[79] Cooper JF, Leadbetter WF, Chute R. The thoracoabdominal approach for retroperitoneal
     gland dissection: its application to testis tumor. J Am Coll Surg (Surg Gynecol Obstet) 1950;
     90:486.
[80] Donohue JP. Retroperitoneal lymphadenectomy: the anterior approach including bilateral
     suprahilar dissection. Urol Clin North Am 1977;4:509.
[81] Richie JP. Modified retroperitoneal lymphadenectomy for patients with clinical stage
     I testicular cancer. Semin Urol 1988;6:216–22.
[82] Jewett MA, Kong YS, Goldberg SD, et al. Retroperitoneal lymphadenectomy for testis
     tumor with nerve sparing for ejaculation. J Urol 1988;139(6):1220–4.
[83] Donohue JP, Foster RS, Rowland RG, et al. Nerve-sparing retroperitoneal lymphadenec-
     tomy with preservation of ejaculation. J Urol 1990;144(2 Pt 1):287–91.
[84] Donohue JP, Thornhill JA, Foster RS, et al. Retroperitoneal lymphadenectomy for clinical
     stage A testis cancer (1965 to 1989): modifications of technique and impact on ejaculation.
     J Urol 1993;149(2):237.
[85] Coogan CL, Hejase MJ, Wahle GR, et al. Nerve sparing post-chemotherapy retroperitoneal
     lymph node dissection for advanced testicular cancer. J Urol 1996;156:1656.
[86] Steiner H, Peschel R, Janetschek G, et al. Long-term results of laparoscopic retroperitoneal
     lymph node dissection: a single-center 10-year experience. Urology 2004;63(3):550–5.
[87] Hara I, Kawabata G, Yamada Y, et al. Extraperitoneal laparoscopic retroperitoneal lymph
     node dissection in supine position after chemotherapy for advanced testicular carcinoma.
     Int J Urol 2004;11(10):934–9.

ELSEVIER
SAUNDERS

Surg Oncol Clin N Am
14 (2005) 569–586

SURGICAL
ONCOLOGY CLINICS
OF NORTH AMERICA

Abdominoperineal Resection for Rectal Cancer: Historic Perspective and Current Issues

David B. Chessin, MD[a],
Jose G. Guillem, MD, MPH[b,c,*]

[a]*Colorectal Service, Department of Surgery, Memorial Sloan-Kettering Cancer Center,
1275 York Avenue, Room C-1083, New York, NY 10021, USA*
[b]*Colorectal Service, Department of Surgery, Memorial Sloan-Kettering Cancer Center,
1275 York Avenue, Room C-1077, New York, NY 10021, USA*
[c]*Cornell University Medical College, 520 East 70th Street, New York, NY 10021, USA*

Rectal cancer continues to be an important health care issue in the United States, affecting an estimated 40,570 people in 2004 [1]. In addition to being a significant cause of mortality, inadequately treated rectal cancer can result in symptoms that are troublesome and difficult to eradicate. Although locally advanced disease is frequently treated with a combination of radiation and chemotherapy, surgical resection remains an essential component of the multimodality treatment of this disease. Among the numerous surgical options for removal of a rectal cancer, the abdominoperineal resection (APR) is considered the most radical, as it results in a permanent colostomy. Our aim is to provide an historic perspective on the development of the APR and review the current issues and indications related to this procedure.

Historic perspective

During the late nineteenth and early twentieth century, most distal rectal cancer presented with advanced, symptomatic disease, and was treated with perineal proctectomy [2]. Patients were treated with a two-stage operation: the first stage included abdominal exploration for metastases and creation of

* Corresponding author. Memorial Sloan-Kettering Cancer Center, 1275 York Avenue, Room C-1077, New York, NY 10021.
E-mail address: guillemj@mskcc.org (J.G. Guillem).

1055-3207/05/$ - see front matter © 2005 Elsevier Inc. All rights reserved.
doi:10.1016/j.soc.2005.04.002 *surgonc.theclinics.com*

Box 1. Rectal cancer surgical milestones

1776: Pillore performs a cecostomy for an obstructing rectal cancer [4]

1826: Lisfranc performs what is believed to be the first excision of rectal cancer

1884: Czerny performs what is believed to be the first combined abdominal and perineal resection of the rectum

1885: Kraske performs trans-sacral rectal resection [5]

1892: Maunsell reports "a new method of excising the two upper portions of the rectum" [6]

1896: Chalot and Quenu first report planned APR of the rectum [7,8]

1899: Waldeyer and Harman describe the anatomy of the pelvic autonomic nerves [9,10]

1908: Miles reports his method of APR [11]

1928: Rankin develops technique for anterior resection [12]

1939: Lloyd-Davies popularizes the two-team approach and lithotomy-Trendelenburg position for APR [13]

1948: Dixon reports a large series of patients who underwent anterior resection and sutured bowel anastomosis [14]

1951: Deddish introduces the concept of extended lateral pelvic lymphadenectomy [15]

1952: Grinnell encourages high ligation of the IMA [16]

1959: Introduction of mechanical bowel preparation

1963: Turell reports on the clinical introduction of fiberoptic endoscopy [17]

1966: Ravitch and Rivarola report the use of surgical staplers for gastrointestinal anastomosis [18]

1970: York Mason reports his technique of transsphincteric rectal resection [19]

1972: Parks reports hand-sewn coloanal anastomosis [20]

1973: Lee, Maurer, and Block report rectal resection with pelvic autonomic nerve preservation [21]

1980: Knight and Griffen report the double-stapled technique of LAR [22]

1982: Heald popularizes the concept of total mesorectal excision [23]

1982: Hojo revisits extended lateral pelvic lymphadenectomy [24]

1984: Buess publishes initial report of transanal endoscopic microsurgery [25]

1984: Shukla and Hughes report perineal wound reconstruction with RAM flap following APR [26]

1986: Quirke documents the importance of the circumferential
margin in local failure [27]
1986: Beynon provides clinical model of endorectal ultrasound
imaging of rectal cancer [28]
1986: Lazorthes and Parc introduce the coloanal J-pouch-anal
anastomosis [29,30]
1992: Sackier et al. report first laparoscopic APR [31]
1997: Z'Graggen introduces the transverse coloplasty-anal
anastomosis [32]

Abbreviations: APR, abdominoperineal resection; LAR, low anterior resection;
IMA, inferior mesenteric artery; RAM flap, rectus abdominus myocutaneous flap.

a left iliac loop sigmoid colostomy, followed in approximately 2 weeks by
perineal resection of the rectum, and in many cases the levator ani muscles
and coccyx [3]. Unfortunately, this procedure was associated with extremely
high morbidity and local recurrence rates up to 100% in many series. In this
setting, the APR for rectal cancer was developed (Box 1).

As early as 1878, Von Volkmann [33,34] discussed the potential utility of
a combined abdominal and perineal approach to rectal cancer, but felt the
operation was contraindicated due to the prohibitive potential for serious
infectious complications. It is believed that Vincent Czerny performed the
first combined abdominal and perineal resection of the rectum in 1884
[11,35]. However, Czerny performed this unplanned procedure after not
being able to complete the rectal resection from a perineal approach [35].
In 1896, the French surgeons Chalot and Quenu each published reports of
planned APR [7,8]. In addition, in 1903, Charles Mayo reported his
experience with a combined abdominal and perineal approach for rectal
cancer, during which time he would perform a laparotomy for exploration,
with the option of a palliative colostomy if the rectal cancer was deemed
unresectable [36]. However, the abdominoperineal approach was not widely
practiced until the publication of the landmark work of William Ernest
Miles, in 1908, entitled "A Method of Performing Abdomino-Perineal
Excision for Carcinoma of the Rectum and Terminal Portion of the Pelvic
Colon" [11].

Dr. Miles, concerned about his prohibitively high local failure rate
following perineal resection of rectal cancer (54 of 57 of his patients failed
within 3 years of follow-up), critically reviewed his personal surgical
experience with this disease (Fig. 1) [11]. He felt that the excessive recurrence
rate was due, in large part, to inadequate lymphadenectomy. This theory
was later supported by autopsy studies, as well as a pathologic study by
Gabriel from St. Marks Hospital in which proximal lymph node metastases
were identified in 56% of patients with rectal cancer [37,38].

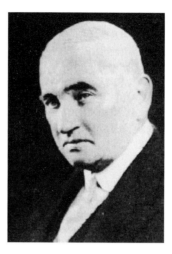

Fig. 1. W.E. Miles (1869–1947). (*From* Wiley MJ, Rieger N. Audit and the birth of the abdomino-perineal excision for carcinoma of the rectum. ANZ J Surg 2003;73:858–61; with permission.)

In response to this uniformly poor oncologic outcome, Miles developed an improved technique to surgically resect the primary tumor and the potentially involved proximal and distal lymph nodes. The Miles' APR involved radical resection of the lymphatics that drain the rectum, including the "zone of upward spread" (along the rectosigmoid mesentery), the levator ani muscle, the ischiorectal fat, and the perineal skin (Fig. 2). Although his procedure was associated with a high mortality (5 of his first 12 patients died postoperatively), three patients survived 4 years without recurrence [39].

Controversy over proximal vascular ligation

As described by Miles, the inferior mesenteric artery (IMA) was ligated just distal to the takeoff of the left colic artery when performing an APR. However, as early as 1908, surgeons such as Moynihan encouraged ligation of the IMA near its origin because of the theoretic advantage that it would provide for more radical clearance of lymphatic tissue potentially involved with tumor [11,40]. This view was supported by the work of Grinnell and Bacon during the 1950s, that demonstrated that lymph nodes near the origin of the IMA were involved with tumor in 11% to 17% of patients with rectal cancer [16,41]. Therefore, Grinnell championed high ligation of the IMA in an attempt to provide for more radical clearance of potentially involved lymphatic tissue [16]. However, it was later documented that there was little benefit to this approach, as there was no improvement in 5-year survival when patients with rectal cancer treated with arterial ligation proximal to the origin of the left colic artery (high ligation) were compared with those treated with arterial ligation distal to the origin of the left colic artery (low

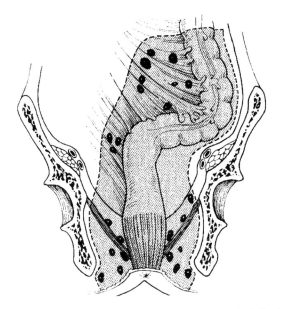

Fig. 2. Extent of abdominoperineal resection, as described by W.E. Miles in his landmark paper in 1908. Demonstrated is what Miles felt were potential sites for tumor involvement, including involvement of extramural tissue distal to the primary tumor and below the levator ani muscle, including the ischiorectal fossa. (*From* Miles WE. A method for performing abdominoperineal excision for carcinoma of the rectum and of the terminal portion of the pelvic colon. Lancet 1908;2:1812–3; with permission.)

ligation) [42]. Currently, as involvement of lymph nodes proximal to the left colic artery is likely a marker of disseminated disease and patients are unlikely to derive oncologic benefit from high arterial ligation, most surgeons ligate the IMA just distal to the takeoff of the left colic artery when performing an APR.

Improvement in morbidity and mortality following abdominoperineal resection

Although associated with a significant improvement in long-term oncologic outcome, the Miles APR was fraught with a high early postoperative mortality rate. The innovation of the two-team approach to APR in 1934 and the clinical availability of blood transfusion in 1939 substantially reduced the mortality associated with this procedure [43]. However, high postoperative morbidity rates, including significant genitourinary and sexual dysfunction, lead to substantial impairment in quality of life following APR.

Another difficult management issue following APR was related to the permanent colostomy, largely due to the lack of durable, high-quality, ostomy care products and limited patient education and support by trained enterostomal therapists. Although Daguesceau reported the first ostomy appliance in 1795, it was not until 1954 that the field of modern stoma therapy was initiated by Dr. Rupert Turnbull and his patient, a nurse named Norma Gill [44]. Dr. Turnbull created a permanent ileostomy as part of his treatment of Ms. Gill's ulcerative colitis, and she became active in assisting others with ostomies. In 1958, Dr. Turnbull hired her as the first enterostomal therapist, and in 1961, they opened the first school for enterostomal therapy. Since that time, advances in ostomy education and technology have substantially improved the quality of life for patients treated with an APR and permanent colostomy.

A change in surgical technique: emphasis on sphincter preservation and total mesorectal excision

During the 1950s to 1970s, outcome following APR for rectal cancer remained stable, with local recurrence rates of 38% and 5-year overall survival of 47% to 52% reported in large series [45,46]. Through this period, we witnessed the development of the coloanal anastomosis by Parks in 1972, and the double-stapled technique of low anterior resection (LAR) by Knight and Griffen in 1980, which resulted in a decrease in the number of patients treated with APR [20,22]. However, local failure rates following APR for rectal cancer remained as high as 37% into the early 1980s [47,48]. In 1984, Shukla and Hughes [26] reported the utility of the rectus abdominus myocutaneous (RAM) flap for perineal reconstruction following APR in an effort to decrease the rate of perineal complications.

In 1982, Heald popularized the concept of total mesorectal excision (TME) in an attempt to reduce the local recurrence rate following resection of rectal cancer. The impact of TME and its associated reduction in positive circumferential resection margin (CRM) rates and local recurrence after resection of rectal cancer was demonstrated by Heald in 1986 and Enker in 1995 [49,50], who reported local recurrence rates of 5% and 7%, respectively. In 1986, Quirke [27] provided pathologic support for optimal resection and its impact on local recurrence rates when he documented a significantly increased rate of local recurrence in rectal cancer patients with a positive CRM.

Current issues surrounding abdominoperineal resection

Important issues related to APR include continued improvement in long-term oncologic outcome using total mesorectal excision, with close attention to obtaining negative proximal, distal, and circumferential resection margins, while preserving the pelvic autonomic nerves, resulting in improved postoperative genitourinary and sexual function and quality of life. Other current issues pertaining to APR include the appropriate use of laparoscopy, as well as the indications and timing for chemoradiation. In the sections that follow, these important issues, as well as the indications for APR, are discussed.

Total mesorectal excision

The mesorectum consists of the fatty tissue surrounding the rectum, which contains small nerves, blood vessels, lymphatic vessels, and lymph nodes. TME is a technique that requires precise dissection in an areolar plane between the visceral fascia that envelops the rectum and mesorectum and the parietal fascia overlying the pelvic wall structures. Critical analysis of the outcome of TME-based APR is somewhat difficult, as most of the available reports are of heterogeneous study groups containing both APR and sphincter-preserving resections.

However, in a study limited to patients with Dukes B and C rectal cancer treated with APR with TME, a 5-year overall survival of 60% and a local recurrence rate of 13% were reported [43]. Of note, nearly half of these patients received pelvic radiation. These results compare favorably to overall survival rates of 31% and local recurrence rates of 37% reported for rectal cancer treated with APR and conventional surgical resection [47,51]. Thus, it appears that a TME-based APR for rectal cancer provides for superior oncologic results when compared with a conventional APR.

Circumferential resection margin

The CRM (also known as the lateral margin) is defined as the distance from the outermost part of the tumor or tumor deposit to the lateral resection margin [27]. In 1986, Quirke and colleagues [27] first reported that a positive CRM is significantly associated with local recurrence after curative rectal cancer resection. Others later corroborated this finding, reporting that a positive CRM is associated with a 3.5-fold to 12-fold increased risk of local recurrence and a 2-fold to 3.7-fold increased risk of death [52–57]. On multivariate analysis, a CRM <1 mm has been reported as an independent predictor of local recurrence [57]. Therefore, the surgeon must make all efforts to obtain a CRM >1 mm when resecting a rectal cancer, including en bloc resection of contiguous structures. The detailed attention to obtaining an appropriate CRM is likely to contribute to decreased rates of local recurrence, distant metastases, and death.

Autonomic nerve preservation

The pelvic autonomic nerves are intimately involved with genitourinary and sexual function. In 1899, Waldeyer and Harman first reported the complexity of the pelvic splanchnic nerves [9,10]. However, it was not until years later that their importance in sexual dysfunction following radical rectal resection was first reported [58]. The sympathetic nerves of the pelvis originate from the T12 to L3 ventral nerve roots, ultimately forming the preaortic superior hypogastric plexus (Fig. 3) [59,60]. Distal to the aortic bifurcation, the superior hypogastric plexus gives rise to the right and left hypogastric nerves, which are closely approximated to the visceral fascia of the mesorectum. They are involved in ejaculation, orgasm, and urinary continence [60]. Injury to the hypogastric sympathetic nerve trunks results in increased bladder tone with reduced bladder capacity, voiding difficulty, impaired ejaculation in men, and loss of vaginal lubrication and dyspareunia in women.

The parasympathetic nerves of the pelvis (nervi erigentes), arise from the S2, S3, and S4 ventral nerves roots (Fig. 3) [59,60]. They are involved in erectile function, vaginal lubrication, and innervation of the detrusor muscle of the bladder [60]. Damage to the parasympathetic nerves leads to erectile dysfunction, impaired vaginal lubrication, and voiding difficulty. The nervi erigentes (parasympathetic) join the hypogastric nerves (sympathetic) on the pelvic sidewall to form the inferior hypogastric plexus (pelvic autonomic nerve plexus), located posterolateral to the seminal vesicles [59,60].

APR has been reported to be associated with a higher rate of sexual dysfunction when compared with patients treated with a LAR [61]. In fact, a large report documented preservation of sexual function following

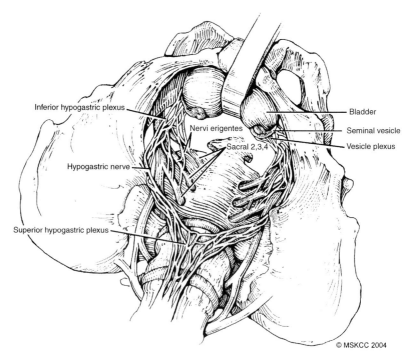

Fig. 3. Pelvic autonomic nerve anatomy. (Courtesy of Memorial Sloan Kettering Cancer Center.)

autonomic nerve preservation (ANP) in 86% of patients undergoing LAR, significantly better than the 57% reported for patients undergoing APR ($P < .05$) [43]. It must be emphasized, however, that factors other than ANP, such as use of chemoradiation, patient comorbidities (ie, atherosclerosis, diabetes mellitus, hypertension), medications (ie, beta-blockers), alcohol use, and age of the patient may contribute to genitourinary and sexual dysfunction following radical rectal resection. Currently, performing an APR according to the principles of TME with ANP can provide for optimal oncologic outcome with maintenance of sexual and urinary function in the majority of patients. In addition, a recent report suggested that the rate of sexual dysfunction may be further reduced by using intraoperative nerve stimulators to help identify and preserve the pelvic autonomic nerves [62].

Oncologic outcome following abdominoperineal resection

Most series report that patients with rectal cancer treated with APR have a worse oncologic outcome when compared with those treated with a sphincter-preserving radical resection (Table 1). A recent prospective report of a large cohort of patients with rectal cancer undergoing resection according to the principals of TME suggests that patients with tumors less than 5 cm from the anal verge (and thus more likely to require APR) have a worse oncologic outcome. This was due, in large part, to the increased incidence of T4 tumors, intraoperative bowel perforation, and positive CRM in these distal tumors [63]. From this report and others, it appears that distal rectal cancers requiring an APR present with more locally advanced disease and poorer pathologic features than cancers in the proximal rectum [43,50]. Also, distal rectal cancers have lymphatic drainage

Table 1
Retrospective series comparing of oncologic outcome for rectal cancer treated with open APR versus LAR

Study (year)	N	F/U (months)	LR-APR (%)	LR-LAR (%)	P	OS-APR (%)	OS-LAR (%)	P
Enker 1997 [43]	APR = 148 LAR = 170	NR	13	NR	NR	60	81	<.0003
Lavery 1997 [66]	APR = 99 LAR = 162	APR = 61 LAR = 70	11	8	.41	62	71	.2
Heald 1997 [69]	APR = 31 LAR = 105	92	47	4	NR	29	68	NR
Jatzko 1999 [64]	APR = 124 LAR = 411	59	16	11	.05	57	71	.001
Wibe 2004 [63]	APR = 821 LAR = 1315	44	15	10	.008	55	68	<.001

Abbreviations: APR, abdominoperineal resection; F/U, follow-up; LAR, low anterior resection; LR, local recurrence; NR, not reported; OS, overall survival.

that allows access to both the portal and systemic circulation, which can results in a higher incidence of distant metastatic disease.

Using a multivariate analysis, a recent large series suggested T and N stage, distance of tumor from the anal verge, intraoperative bowel perforation, and positive CRM correlated with local recurrence, while procedure performed (LAR versus APR) did not [63,64]. The oncologic outcome for rectal cancer of similar stage, pathologic features, and distance from the anal verge treated with APR does not appear to be different from those treated with LAR, provided the resection is performed with meticulous surgical technique according to the principals of TME [63,65–68]. Therefore, it appears that patients with distal rectal cancer requiring APR may have a poorer long-term oncologic outcome related more to anatomic and tumor factors, and perhaps less on the procedure performed.

Because extramural involvement distal to the rectal cancer and below the levator ani muscles is rare (Fig. 4), dissection below the levator ani muscle and resection of the ischiorectal tissue, as advocated by Miles to address distal tumor deposits (Fig. 2), may not be oncologically necessary unless there is direct involvement by the primary tumor [69]. This is supported by a recent report of 136 patients treated with TME (and no preoperative

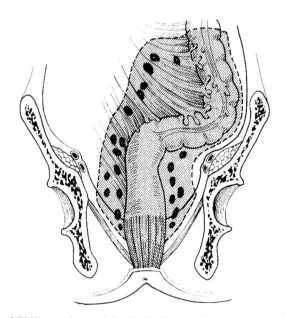

Fig. 4. Extent of TME, as advocated by Heald. Illustrated is the region of potential nodal involvement from a primary rectal cancer. Note that involvement of lymph nodes distal to the primary tumor and below the levator ani muscle is considered to be extremely rate. Thus, if there is no direct tumor extension, this tissue is not routinely resected. (*From* Heald RJ, Smedh RK, Kald A, et al. Abdominoperineal excision of the rectum—an endangered operation. Norman Nigro Lectureship. Dis Colon Rectum 1997;40:747–51; with permission.)

chemotherapy or radiation) that documented a local recurrence below the levators (perineal wound or scar) of 10% after APR compared with a local recurrence rate of 1% after curative LAR [69]. These results prompted Heald [69] to conclude that the perineal wound itself "may be a pre-requisite for local perineal recurrence" following curative resection of distal rectal cancer and that an APR should rarely be performed. These conclusions must be interpreted carefully, as they are based on a small sample size (n = 31 APR) and the fact that none of these patients received preoperative radiation therapy, which would have limited viable tumor shedding and perineal wound recurrence during resection of bulky tumors. We feel that an APR still has an important role in the treatment of properly selected patients with rectal cancer.

Quality of life

Postoperative quality of life is a major concern following APR for rectal cancer. A recent, prospective study using the EORTC QLQ-30 and CR-38 questionnaires documented that patients with rectal cancer undergoing LAR have improved quality of life when compared with patients undergoing APR. In addition, patients who had no stoma, or had their stoma reversed, had a substantially improved postoperative quality of life compared with patients with a permanent stoma [70]. However, another large series, using the same questionnaires, reported opposite results. Patients with a permanent stoma reported significantly better social function ($P = .005$), less anxiety ($P = .008$), and higher self-esteem ($P = .0002$) than patients who underwent restoration of bowel continuity [71]. These latter findings have been supported by others in the literature [72].

It is clear that postoperative quality of life is dependent upon the interaction of patient factors (ie, age, gender, comorbidities, and pre-operative anorectal function), tumor factors (ie, extent of local invasion), and treatment/surgical factors (ie, use of preoperative chemoradiation, level of the anastomosis, use of intraoperative radiation therapy) [61,73,74]. Therefore, because of the multiplicity of factors involved, more sensitive, validated instruments to evaluate quality of life following APR are required.

Laparoscopic surgery

Laparoscopic APR, first reported by Sackier in 1992, may provide for decreased postoperative pain, earlier return of bowel function, and a shorter hospital stay when compared with open rectal resection [31,75–77]. In addition, it is anticipated that direct vision deep within the pelvis using magnified, angled optics may be especially beneficial for performing an APR with ANP in obese male patients with a narrow pelvis. However, whether these potential benefits translate into improved patient outcome remains to be confirmed, as the only data concerning laparoscopic APR for rectal cancer is from small, nonrandomized series.

Be that as it may, the available reports suggest that laparoscopic-assisted APR for rectal cancer is feasible, with acceptable short-term morbidity and postoperative mortality, when performed by experienced surgeons [76–78]. The overall postoperative morbidity has been reported between 6% to 44% for laparoscopic APR, compared with 28% to 66% for open APR [75–77]. In addition, operative blood loss, return of bowel function, and hospital stay have been reported to be reduced when the laparoscopic-assisted approach is compared with open APR [75,79,80]. Most importantly, recent reports suggest that oncologic outcome is not compromised by laparoscopic-assisted APR [76,79]. When the principals of TME are followed by experienced surgeons, local recurrence rates of 4% to 21%, 5-year disease-specific survival of 75% to 92%, and 5-year overall survival of 65% to 100% have been reported with laparoscopic rectal cancer resection [79,80,81]. In addition, it appears that margin status and number of lymph nodes retrieved is not impaired when the laparoscopic approach is used by experienced surgeons [75,81].

Although the available data is encouraging, it is difficult to conclusively evaluate laparoscopic APR in terms of long-term local control and survival, as the available studies are heterogeneous with regard to tumor stage and use of neoadjuvant and adjuvant therapy. Also, to date, patients with rectal cancer have been excluded from all prospective, randomized trials of laparoscopic versus open resection, in large part, because of the complexity of rectal resection and difficulty in assessing quality control of TME. As such, we await the results of large, prospective, randomized trials before definitive recommendations can be made concerning the safety and oncologic efficacy of laparoscopic APR for rectal cancer.

The role of chemoradiation in the setting of an abdominoperineal resection

A recently reported prospective, randomized trial comparing preoperative and postoperative chemoradiation (50.4 Gy of external beam pelvic radiation and 5-fluorouracil-based chemotherapy) for locally advanced rectal cancer demonstrated the superiority of the preoperative regimen with regards to local control and sphincter preservation rates [82]. However, the study included a heterogeneous group of patients treated with either APR or sphincter-preserving techniques. Another prospective, randomized trial comparing the use of short-course preoperative radiation therapy (5 Gy over 5 days) and TME to TME alone for the treatment of rectal cancer (including both APR and sphincter-preserving resection) documented a significantly decreased 2-year local recurrence rate for patients treated with preoperative radiation therapy (2.4% versus 8.2%, $P < .001$) [83]. The results of this study must be interpreted carefully, however, in that the available pathologic quality control data suggests that up to 24% of patients had a suboptimal TME and a higher than expected 23% of patients had a positive resection margin [84]. Of note, it appears that pelvic irradiation in patients with a suboptimal CRM (less than 1 mm) does not improve local recurrence rates, emphasizing the importance of surgical resection and negative resection margins on oncologic outcome [85].

In addition to the oncologic advantages of preoperative chemoradiation for patients with rectal cancer, this approach avoids irradiating the colorectal anastomosis and small bowel that may become fixed in the pelvis following resection. However, this must be balanced against the potential for increased perineal wound morbidity, reported in 7% to 66% of patients treated with preoperative radiation followed by APR [86]. Procedures such as the RAM flap can be used to significantly decrease perineal wound morbidity following an APR. However, the perineal defect remains a significant consideration when planning preoperative chemoradiation for a rectal cancer requiring APR [86].

It is reasonable to suggest that properly selected patients may benefit from preoperative therapy, even when the rectal cancer is resected using TME. Currently, we advocate preoperative chemoradiation for locally advanced rectal cancer (endorectal ultrasound T3–4 or N1 or clinically bulky). In the future, it is anticipated that imaging modalities such as endorectal ultrasound, MRI, CT, and positron emission tomography may be used to optimally select patients for treatment with chemoradiation [87–89].

Indications for abdominoperineal resection

Even though APR was first introduced over a century ago, it still accounts for 18% to 27% of the surgical procedures performed for rectal adenocarcinoma, and remains an important technique in the surgical management of this disease [48,83,90,91]. Absolute indications for APR include involvement of the levator ani muscle or inability to resect a large tumor with negative CRM via an isolated abdominal approach (Box 2).

Other indications for APR include persistent or recurrent anal squamous cancer and rare anal tumors (adenocarcinoma, melanoma, carcinoid,

---

Box 2. Indications for abdominoperineal resection

Rectal adenocarcinoma involving the levator ani muscle
Inability to resect distal rectal adenocarcinoma with negative
    margins via the abdominal approach alone
Persistent or recurrent anal squamous cancer
Bulky pelvic tumor recurrence
Rare tumors of the anus (ie, adenocarcinoma, melanoma,
    carcinoid, sarcoma, others) too large to be managed with local
    procedures alone
Chordoma involving the levator ani muscle

sarcoma, and others) that involve the sphincters or are too large to be adequately treated with local excision. Also, chordoma or other rare pelvic tumors involving the levator ani muscles may be treated with an APR. In addition, bulky pelvic recurrences, that may or may not involve the sphincters, often require a combined abdominal and perineal approach to ensure a resection with negative CRM.

Summary

The technique of APR has changed substantially in the past century, with significant improvements in early postoperative outcome, long-term oncologic outcome, and quality of life. APR, according to the principles of TME, has provided for substantial improvement in local failure and overall survival rates. In addition, when oncologically appropriate, APR performed with ANP can contribute to substantial improvements in postoperative genitourinary and sexual function. Experience with laparoscopic-assisted APR suggests that this procedure may provide for decreased postoperative morbidity, and appears safe and effective for rectal cancer resection. However, large, prospective studies are needed before definitive conclusions can be drawn.

The future challenges in the management of a patient with rectal cancer felt to require an APR include the determination of the optimal use of chemoradiation and immunologic therapy, better definition of the role of laparoscopy, better understanding of the pathophysiology of bladder and sexual dysfunction, and further improvement in local and distant control of disease. It is important to recognize that a century after its introduction, APR remains a valuable procedure in the curative treatment of select patients with distal rectal tumors.

References

[1] Jemal A, Tiwari RC, Murray T, et al. Cancer statistics, 2004. CA Cancer J Clin 2004;54:8–29.
[2] Lockhardt-Mummery J. Two hundred cases of cancer of the rectum treated by perineal excision. Br J Surg 1926;14:110–24.
[3] Ruo L, Guillem JG. Major 20th-century advancements in the management of rectal cancer. Dis Colon Rectum 1999;42:563–78.
[4] Pillore H. Opération d'anus artificiel, pratiquée en 1776. Expér J Méd Chir 1840;5:73.
[5] Kraske P. Zur exstirpation hoch sitzender mastdarmkrebske. Verh Dtsch Ges Chir 1985;14:464–74.
[6] Maunsell H. A new method of excising the two upper portions of the rectum and the lower segment of the sigmoid flexure of the colon. Lancet 1892;2:473–6.
[7] Chalot V. Nouvelle méthode abdomino-périnéale pour l'extirpation totale de l'anus, du rectum et, au besoin, de l'S iliaqu cancereux, avec colostomie iliaque. Bull Mem Soc Chir Paris 1896:310–8.
[8] Quenu M. Traitement du cancer du rectum; procède nouveau d'extirpation totale abdomino-périnéale. Bull Mem Soc Chir Paris 1896:270–85.

[9] Waldeyer W. Das Becken. In: Cohen F, editor. Bonn; 1899.
[10] Harman N. The pelvic splanchnic nerves. J Anat Physiol 1899;33:386–99.
[11] Miles WE. A method for performing abdominoperineal excision for carcinoma of the rectum and of the terminal portion of the pelvic colon. Lancet 1908;2:1812–3.
[12] Rankin F. The technique of anterior resection of the rectosigmoid. Surg Gynecol Obstet 1928;46:537–46.
[13] Lloyd-Davies O. Lithotomy-Trendelenburg position for resection of the rectum and lower pelvic colon. Lancet 1939;2:74.
[14] Dixon C. Anterior resection for malignant lesions of the upper part of the rectum and lower part of the sigmoid. Ann Surg 1948;128:425–42.
[15] Deddish MR. Abdominopelvic lymphnode dissection in cancer of the rectum and distal colon. Cancer 1951;4:1364–6.
[16] Grinnell RS, Hiatt RB. Ligation of the interior mesenteric artery at the aorta in resections for carcinoma of the sigmoid and rectum. Surg Gynecol Obstet 1952;94:526–34.
[17] Turell R. Fiber optic coloscope and sigmoidoscope. Am J Surg 1963;105:133–6.
[18] Ravitch MM, Rivarola A. Enteroanastomosis with an automatic instrument. Surgery 1966;59:270–7.
[19] Mason AY. Surgical access to the rectum—a transsphincteric exposure. Proc R Soc Med 1970;63(Suppl):91–4.
[20] Parks A. Transanal technique in low rectal anastomosis. Proc R Soc Med 1972;65:975–6.
[21] Lee JF, Maurer VM, Block GE. Anatomic relations of pelvic autonomic nerves to pelvic operations. Arch Surg 1973;107:324–8.
[22] Knight CD, Griffen FD. An improved technique for low anterior resection of the rectum using the EEA stapler. Surgery 1980;88:710–4.
[23] Heald RJ, Husband EM, Ryall RD. The mesorectum in rectal cancer surgery—the clue to pelvic recurrence? Br J Surg 1982;69:613–6.
[24] Hojo K, Koyama Y, Moriya Y. Lymphatic spread and its prognostic value in patients with rectal cancer. Am J Surg 1982;144:350–4.
[25] Buess G, Hutterer F, Theiss J, et al. A system for a transanal endoscopic rectum operation. Chirurg 1984;55:677–80.
[26] Shukla HS, Hughes LE. The rectus abdominis flap for perineal wounds. Ann R Coll Surg Engl 1984;66:337–9.
[27] Quirke P, Durdey P, Dixon MF, et al. Local recurrence of rectal adenocarcinoma due to inadequate surgical resection. Histopathological study of lateral tumour spread and surgical excision. Lancet 1986;2:996–9.
[28] Beynon J, Foy DM, Temple LN, et al. The endosonic appearances of normal colon and rectum. Dis Colon Rectum 1986;29:810–3.
[29] Lazorthes F, Fages P, Chiotasso P, et al. Resection of the rectum with construction of a colonic reservoir and colo-anal anastomosis for carcinoma of the rectum. Br J Surg 1986;73:136–8.
[30] Parc R, Tiret E, Frileux P, et al. Resection and colo-anal anastomosis with colonic reservoir for rectal carcinoma. Br J Surg 1986;73:139–41.
[31] Sackier JM, Berci G, Hiatt JR, et al. Laparoscopic abdominoperineal resection of the rectum. Br J Surg 1992;79:1207–8.
[32] Z'Graggen K, Maurer CA, Buchler MW. Transverse coloplasty pouch. A novel neorectal reservoir. Dig Surg 1999;16:363–6.
[33] Von Volkmann R. Ueber den Mastdarmkrebs und die Exstirpatio recti. Samml klin Vortr 1878;131:1113–28.
[34] Corman A. Classic articles in colonic and rectal surgery. Richard von Volkmann 1830–1889. Concerning rectal cancer and the removal of the rectum. Dis Colon Rectum 1986;29:679–85.
[35] Miles WE. A method of performing abdomino-perineal excision for carcinoma of the rectum and of the terminal portion of the pelvic colon (1908). CA Cancer J Clin 1971;21:361–4.

[36] Mayo C. Evolution in the treatment of cancer of the rectum. JAMA 1903;40:1127–9.
[37] Gabriel W. Perineo-abdominal excision of the rectum in one stage. Lancet 1934;2: 69–74.
[38] Wiley MJ, Rieger N. Audit and the birth of the abdomino-perineal excision for carcinoma of the rectum. ANZ J Surg 2003;73:858–61.
[39] Miles WE. The treatment of carcinoma of the rectum and pelvic colon. Glasgow Med J 1912; 2:81–104.
[40] Moynihan B. The surgical treatment of cancer of the sigmoid flexure and rectum. Surg Gynecol Obstet 1908;6:463–6.
[41] Bacon HE, Dirbas F, Myers TB, et al. Extensive lymphad enectomy and high ligation of the inferior mesenteric artery for carcinoma of the left colon and rectum. Dis Colon Rectum 1958;1:457–64 [discussion: 464–5].
[42] Pezim ME, Nicholls RJ. Survival after high or low ligation of the inferior mesenteric artery during curative surgery for rectal cancer. Ann Surg 1984;200:729–33.
[43] Enker WE, Havenga K, Polyak T, et al. Abdominoperineal resection via total mesorectal excision and autonomic nerve preservation for low rectal cancer. World J Surg 1997;21: 715–20.
[44] Cataldo PA. Intestinal stomas: 200 years of digging. Dis Colon Rectum 1999;42:137–42.
[45] Patel SC, Tovee EB, Langer B. Twenty-five years of experience with radical surgical treatment of carcinoma of the extraperitoneal rectum. Surgery 1977;82:460–5.
[46] Slanetz CA Jr, Herter FP, Grinnell RS. Anterior resection versus abdominoperineal resection for cancer of the rectum and rectosigmoid. An analysis of 524 cases. Am J Surg 1972;123:110–7.
[47] Athlin L, Bengtsson NO, Stenling R. Local recurrence and survival after radical resection of rectal carcinoma. Acta Chir Scand 1988;154:225–9.
[48] Adloff M, Arnaud JP, Schloegel M, et al. Factors influencing local recurrence after abdominoperineal resection for cancer of the rectum. Dis Colon Rectum 1985;28:413–5.
[49] Heald RJ, Ryall RD. Recurrence and survival after total mesorectal excision for rectal cancer. Lancet 1986;1:1479–82.
[50] Enker WE, Thaler HT, Cranor ML, et al. Total mesorectal excision in the operative treatment of carcinoma of the rectum. J Am Coll Surg 1995;181:335–46.
[51] Rosen L, Veidenheimer MC, Coller JA, et al. Mortality, morbidity, and patterns of recurrence after abdominoperineal resection for cancer of the rectum. Dis Colon Rectum 1982;25:202–8.
[52] Birbeck KF, Macklin CP, Tiffin NJ, et al. Rates of circumferential resection margin involvement vary between surgeons and predict outcomes in rectal cancer surgery. Ann Surg 2002;235:449–57.
[53] Adam IJ, Mohamdee MO, Martin IG, et al. Role of circumferential margin involvement in the local recurrence of rectal cancer. Lancet 1994;344:707–11.
[54] Ng IO, Luk IS, Yuen ST, et al. Surgical lateral clearance in resected rectal carcinomas. A multivariate analysis of clinicopathologic features. Cancer 1993;71:1972–6.
[55] de Haas-Kock DF, Baeten CG, Jager JJ, et al. Prognostic significance of radial margins of clearance in rectal cancer. Br J Surg 1996;83:781–5.
[56] Compton C, Fenoglio-Preiser CM, Pettigrew N, et al. American Joint Committee on Cancer Prognostic Factors Consensus Conference: Colorectal Working Group. Cancer 2000;88: 1739–57.
[57] Wibe A, Rendedal PR, Svensson E, et al. Prognostic significance of the circumferential resection margin following total mesorectal excision for rectal cancer. Br J Surg 2002;89: 327–34.
[58] Jones T. Complications of one stage abdominoperineal resection of the rectum. JAMA 1942; 120:104–7.
[59] Havenga K, Enker WE. Autonomic nerve preserving total mesorectal excision. Surg Clin North Am 2002;82:1009–18.

[60] Havenga K, Maas CP, DeRuiter MC, et al. Avoiding long-term disturbance to bladder and sexual function in pelvic surgery, particularly with rectal cancer. Semin Surg Oncol 2000;18: 235–43.

[61] Havenga K, Enker WE, McDermott K, et al. Male and female sexual and urinary function after total mesorectal excision with autonomic nerve preservation for carcinoma of the rectum. J Am Coll Surg 1996;182:495–502.

[62] Hanna NN, Guillem J, Dosoretz A, et al. Intraoperative parasympathetic nerve stimulation with tumescence monitoring during total mesorectal excision for rectal cancer. J Am Coll Surg 2002;195:506–12.

[63] Wibe A, Syse A, Andersen E, et al. Oncological outcomes after total mesorectal excision for cure for cancer of the lower rectum: anterior vs. abdominoperineal resection. Dis Colon Rectum 2004;47:48–58.

[64] Jatzko GR, Jagoditsch M, Lisborg PH, et al. Long-term results of radical surgery for rectal cancer: multivariate analysis of prognostic factors influencing survival and local recurrence. Eur J Surg Oncol 1999;25:284–91.

[65] Holm T, Rutqvist LE, Johansson H, et al. Abdominoperineal resection and anterior resection in the treatment of rectal cancer: results in relation to adjuvant preoperative radiotherapy. Br J Surg 1995;82:1213–6.

[66] Lavery IC, Lopez-Kostner F, Fazio VW, et al. Chances of cure are not compromised with sphincter-saving procedures for cancer of the lower third of the rectum. Surgery 1997;122: 779–84 [discussion: 784–5].

[67] Bokey EL, Chapuis PH, Dent OF, et al. Factors affecting survival after excision of the rectum for cancer: a multivariate analysis. Dis Colon Rectum 1997;40:3–10.

[68] Dehni N, McFadden N, McNamara DA, et al. Oncologic results following abdominoperineal resection for adenocarcinoma of the low rectum. Dis Colon Rectum 2003;46:867–74 [discussion: 874].

[69] Heald RJ, Smedh RK, Kald A, et al. Abdominoperineal excision of the rectum—an endangered operation. Norman Nigro Lectureship. Dis Colon Rectum 1997;40:747–51.

[70] Engel J, Kerr J, Schlesinger-Raab A, et al. Quality of life in rectal cancer patients: a four-year prospective study. Ann Surg 2003;238:203–13.

[71] Rauch P, Miny J, Conroy T, et al. Quality of life among disease-free survivors of rectal cancer. J Clin Oncol 2004;22:354–60.

[72] Jess P, Christiansen J, Bech P. Quality of life after anterior resection versus abdominoperineal extirpation for rectal cancer. Scand J Gastroenterol 2002;37:1201–4.

[73] Shibata D, Guillem JG, Lanouette N, et al. Functional and quality-of-life outcomes in patients with rectal cancer after combined modality therapy, intraoperative radiation therapy, and sphincter preservation. Dis Colon Rectum 2000;43:752–8.

[74] Grumann MM, Noack EM, Hoffmann IA, et al. Comparison of quality of life in patients undergoing abdominoperineal extirpation or anterior resection for rectal cancer. Ann Surg 2001;233:149–56.

[75] Wu WX, Sun YM, Hua YB, et al. Laparoscopic versus conventional open resection of rectal carcinoma: a clinical comparative study. World J Gastroenterol 2004;10:1167–70.

[76] Fleshman JW, Wexner SD, Anvari M, et al. Laparoscopic vs. open abdominoperineal resection for cancer. Dis Colon Rectum 1999;42:930–9.

[77] Leung KL, Kwok SP, Lau WY, et al. Laparoscopic-assisted abdominoperineal resection for low rectal adenocarcinoma. Surg Endosc 2000;14:67–70.

[78] Kockerling F, Scheidbach H, Schneider C, et al. Laparoscopic abdominoperineal resection: early postoperative results of a prospective study involving 116 patients. The Laparoscopic Colorectal Surgery Study Group. Dis Colon Rectum 2000;43:1503–11.

[79] Leroy J, Jamali F, Forbes L, et al. Laparoscopic total mesorectal excision (TME) for rectal cancer surgery: long-term outcomes. Surg Endosc 2004;18:281–9.

[80] Morino M, Parini U, Giraudo G, et al. Laparoscopic total mesorectal excision: a consecutive series of 100 patients. Ann Surg 2003;237:335–42.

[81] Feliciotti F, Guerrieri M, Paganini AM, et al. Long-term results of laparoscopic versus open resections for rectal cancer for 124 unselected patients. Surg Endosc 2003;17:1530–5.

[82] Sauer R, Becker H, Hohenberger W, et al. Preoperative versus postoperative chemoradiotherapy for rectal cancer. N Engl J Med 2004;351:1731–40.

[83] Kapiteijn E, Marijnen CA, Nagtegaal ID, et al. Preoperative radiotherapy combined with total mesorectal excision for resectable rectal cancer. N Engl J Med 2001;345:638–46.

[84] Nagtegaal ID, van de Velde CJ, van der Worp E, et al. Macroscopic evaluation of rectal cancer resection specimen: clinical significance of the pathologist in quality control. J Clin Oncol 2002;20:1729–34.

[85] Marijnen CA, Nagtegaal ID, Kapiteijn E, et al. Radiotherapy does not compensate for positive resection margins in rectal cancer patients: report of a multicenter randomized trial. Int J Radiat Oncol Biol Phys 2003;55:1311–20.

[86] Chessin D, Hartley J, Cohen AM, et al. Rectus flap reconstruction decreases perineal wound complications following pelvic chemoradiation and surgery: A Cohort study. Ann Surg Oncol 2005;12(2):104–10.

[87] Guillem JG, Puig-La Calle J Jr, Akhurst T, et al. Prospective assessment of primary rectal cancer response to preoperative radiation and chemotherapy using 18-fluorodeoxyglucose positron emission tomography. Dis Colon Rectum 2000;43:18–24.

[88] Beets-Tan RG, Beets GL, Borstlap AC, et al. Preoperative assessment of local tumor extent in advanced rectal cancer: CT or high-resolution MRI? Abdom Imaging 2000;25:533–41.

[89] Beets-Tan RG, Beets GL, Vliegen RF, et al. Accuracy of magnetic resonance imaging in prediction of tumour-free resection margin in rectal cancer surgery. Lancet 2001;357:497–504.

[90] Martling AL, Holm T, Rutqvist LE, et al. Effect of a surgical training programme on outcome of rectal cancer in the County of Stockholm. Stockholm Colorectal Cancer Study Group, Basingstoke Bowel Cancer Research Project. Lancet 2000;356:93–6.

[91] Nissan A, Guillem JG, Paty PB, et al. Abdominoperineal resection for rectal cancer at a specialty center. Dis Colon Rectum 2001;44:27–35 [discussion: 35–6].

ELSEVIER
SAUNDERS

Surg Oncol Clin N Am
14 (2005) 587–606

SURGICAL
ONCOLOGY CLINICS
OF NORTH AMERICA

Evolution of Pelvic Exenteration

Marvin J. Lopez, MD*, Limaris Barrios, MD

Tufts University School of Medicine, 136 Harrison Avenue, Boston, MA 02111, USA
Department of Surgery, Caritas St. Elizabeth's Medical Center of Boston,
736 Cambridge Street, Boston, MA 01235, USA

Evolution of total pelvic exenteration

Most, if not all, cancer operations as we know them today had been performed successfully by the late 1940s. Surgical advances after World War II, especially in blood transfusion, anesthesia, antibiotic therapy, and later in nutrition and respiratory and intensive care monitoring, made it possible for radical resection procedures such as pancreatoduodenectomy, esophagectomy, radical neck dissection, and abdominoperineal resection of the rectum to become the standard of care in the surgical treatment of malignancy arising from these organs.

Total pelvic exenteration is defined as the complete resection of the pelvic viscera and its draining lymphatic system. Although nearly 60 years have passed since Brunschwig [1] published his initial experience in 1948, the value of this procedure was recognized relatively late in the evolution of radical cancer surgery (Fig. 1). The objective of total pelvic exenteration is to encompass all malignant tissues including adjacent invaded viscera and regional lymphatics; therefore, experience with other pelvic radical cancer operations had to mature for exenterative surgery to have a place in the surgical armamentarium against locally advanced pelvic cancer affecting more than one pelvic organ. These "lesser" procedures include radical cystectomy (Verhoogen, 1908), radical hysterectomy (Weirtheim, 1898), and abdominoperineal rectal resection (Miles, 1908). Each is an extensive surgical procedure capable of inflicting substantial morbidity and functional impairment of great magnitude.

Eugene M. Bricker, a pioneer in pelvic exenteration, performed his first total exenteration on August 8, 1940, at the newly created Ellis Fischel State

---
* Corresponding author. Department of Surgery, Caritas St. Elizabeth's Medical Center of Boston, 736 Cambridge Street, Boston, MA 01235.
E-mail address: Marvin.Lopez.MD@caritaschristi.org (M.J. Lopez).

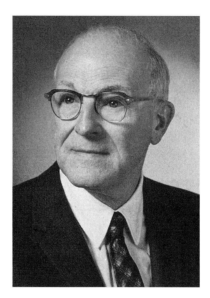

Fig. 1. Alexander Brunschwig, MD. First reported total pelvic exenteration in 1948.

Cancer Hospital in 1939, the first multidisciplinary cancer center west of the Mississippi River (Fig. 2). Bricker's patient was a 32-year-old woman with persistent carcinoma of the uterine cervix. Along with pathologist Lauren Ackerman, radiotherapist Theodore Eberhart (Fig. 3), and Dr. Juan del Regato, Bricker observed that certain cancers arising from the pelvic viscera possessed a propensity for remaining confined to the pelvic organs for long periods before metastasizing beyond the pelvic lymph nodes. Well-differentiated squamous cell carcinoma of the uterine cervix, vagina, and vulva, adenocarcinoma of the rectosigmoid, and visceral and nonvisceral sarcomas were included in this group of cancers. Ovarian, prostatic, and to a lesser extent bladder and endometrial cancers had most often spread beyond the pelvis by the time adjacent viscera were involved. Two decades later, Spratt and associates confirmed these observations [2].

By mid twentieth century, the operation had evolved from an experiment reserved for desperate clinical situations to an established operation. In the hands of a few surgeons, the procedure offered a possibility of cure to selected patients with otherwise incurable advanced pelvic cancer. Thus, by 1960, Brunschwig in New York City, Appleby in Vancouver, BC, Canada, Britnall and Flocks in Iowa City had reported successful experiences with this operation, and Bricker had developed the ileal conduit for urinary diversion, a major advance in pelvic surgery [3]. Improvements in perioperative surgical care, intestinal stoma appliances, radiology, and patient selection made the operation safer. The operative mortality rate declined from over 20% in the period from 1940 to the 1960s, to less than 10% in the 1970s. Continued interest in this subject led to the first

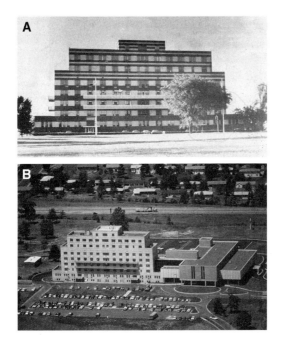

Fig. 2. (*A*) Ellis Fischel Cancer Center, Columbia, MO, 1939. (*B*) Ellis Fischel Cancer Center, Columbia, MO, 1987.

comprehensive publication on exenterative surgery of the pelvis by Spratt and colleagues in 1973 [4]. Subsequently, those of us who were privileged to work for Drs. Bricker and Spratt were inspired to contribute toward making this operation a safe and appropriate option for patients with pelvic cancer that was incurable by other means. As a tribute to them and to the generations of surgeons who follow them, a 50-year institutional experience was reported by our group [5].

The senior author (MJL), who was mentored by Bricker in the late 1970s, witnessed first hand the evolution of an operation during the era of emerging multimodal management of pelvic cancer, including neoadjuvant chemo-radiation therapy, surgical specialty competition for cases requiring the advanced surgery of pelvic malignancy, and improved imaging such as computed tomography, magnetic resonance, and positron emission tomography. Other developments such as prospective randomized clinical trials, evidence-based medicine, advanced laparoscopy, and early cancer detection practices have placed this radical operation in a different perspective. For instance, pelvic exenteration today must be viewed in the context of a salvage operation aimed at a potential cure, not primarily as a palliative effort. Finally, this daunting procedure must be performed by surgeons experienced in multivisceral resections, in an environment in which pelvic reconstruction, patient rehabilitation, and interdisciplinary cancer care are

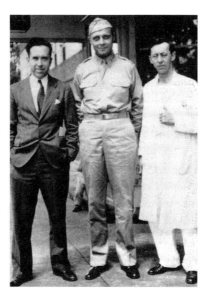

Fig. 3. First multidisciplinary team at Ellis Fischel Cancer Center (from left to right) Drs. Ackerman, Bricker, and Eberhardt.

provided, with the leadership of surgeons who understand and embrace multimodal treatment of patients with cancer.

During the 1990s and the first half of the present decade, total pelvic exenteration has been performed with minimal occurrences of mortality, but the risk of morbidity remains. The reduction of operative mortality rates has permitted surgeons to extend the operation safely to include involved portions of the bony pelvis [6–8]. Although the neglected pelvic cancers commonly observed in decades before early cancer detection practices were performed are now uncommon, pelvic exenteration, with its technical modifications, maintains an important place in the armamentarium against advanced pelvic malignancy. In developing nations, where resources are scarce, multimodal treatment is underused; however, where operative complications are now manageable to the extent of significantly reducing operative mortality, pelvic exenteration is being increasingly used as the primary form of management. Several recent publications attest to the increasing use of this procedure internationally, even in community hospitals [9–12].

This article discusses the surgical results of pelvic exenteration for primary and recurrent rectosigmoid adenocarcinomas, a cancer site that represents the most common clinical scenario and area of interest for general surgeons, surgical oncologists, and colorectal surgeons. Discussion includes the indications for surgery and preoperative evaluation, technique modifications, morbidity, mortality, and survival.

Rationale

The indolent biologic behavior of certain pelvic cancers is what makes pelvic exenteration a feasible procedure for the cure of locally advanced neoplasms. Spratt and Spjut [13] recognized almost 40 years ago that there are rectal cancers associated with good prognoses despite their size. The so-called nonmetastasizing colorectal cancer is characterized by an exophytic morphology, tending toward well-differentiated adenocarcinomas with pushing rather than infiltrating margins; and inflammatory peritumoral reaction is conspicuously absent. These tumors show little propensity for invasion of vascular or lymphatic spaces, and lymph node metastases are infrequent. In current biologic terminology, they tend to be aneuploid, with low DNA content and low S phase fraction, are carcinoembryonic antigen-negative, and show negative p53 proto-oncogene expression. They are, in fact, what some investigators define as "low risk" rectal cancers.

Gall and Hermanek [14] have shown how primitive the current tumor (T) classification is in terms of tumor stage and prognosis after tumor biology is evaluated. In their study, low-risk TNM stage T2 rectal cancers were associated with a 9% lymph node metastatic rate compared with 40% for high-risk T2 tumors. Data have shown that in colorectal cancer, tumor invasion of an adjacent viscera is prognostically more favorable than tumors confined to the bowel wall, with metastases to lymph nodes [15]. Among 86 cases of multivisceral resections for colorectal cancer, more than 80% had histologic evidence of adjacent organ invasion, but in less than 30% were metastases found in the regional lymph nodes. The 5-year survival rate in this group of patients was 76%, despite the locally advanced T stage. Similar findings were reported in a small group of patients treated with total pelvic exenteration for rectal cancer and in another study after resection of portions of the bony pelvis, the so-called composite pelvic exenteration, was performed [6,16].

Understanding the biologic behavior of rectal cancer serves to establish prognostic parameters and treatment planning for patients with recurrent rectal cancer. For primary rectal cancer, the consensus is that high-risk, locally advanced tumors should be treated first with chemo-radiation therapy, with the objective of converting a supraradical operation into a less morbid procedure. Unfortunately, only rarely can chemo-radiation therapy change the indication for pelvic exenteration when it has been envisioned by an experienced pelvic surgeon as the only possible curative surgical intervention.

Indications, contraindications, and patient selection

Pelvic exenteration is indicated as primary or salvage therapy for locally advanced malignancy that has not evidently metastasized outside the anatomical boundaries of the resection. Case selection is paramount to success. If an en-bloc operation of this magnitude has any chance for prolonged disease-free survival or long-term cure, important patient and tumor factors must be taken into account. In this context, it is critical to ascertain how great an impact this operation will have on the physical and mental well being of the patient, which translates into quality of life.

As early as 1950, Bricker [3] stated that "if we are unable to leave a patient in a functional state compatible with a comfortable existence, we are not morally justified in performing this operation." One must be attentive to factors that may have a negative impact on postoperative function, such as the lack of mobility, the inability for self-care, and excessive dependency on others. The sexual incapacitation resulting from this operation must be well understood by the patient and spouse. These social factors must be carefully evaluated in repeated discussions with the patient and family to ensure that all of them understand the implications of the proposed operation.

General preoperative evaluation

Physical factors are easier to evaluate objectively. Although chronologic age offers no categorical barrier, patients older that 70 years generally are not good candidates because most have limited cardiorespiratory reserve. In one recent publication, age was cited as an independent prognostic factor [17]. Significant postoperative morbidity and increased mortality are likely in morbidly obese older patients, poorly controlled diabetics, patients with a history of thromboembolism and intestinal fistulae from previous treatments, and severely malnourished patients. Although none of the above is a strict or categorical contraindication for the operation, a combination of these factors is a contraindication, as is multiorgan dysfunction.

The foremost categorical contraindication for a curative operation is the presence of local or systemic evidence of advanced disease. Progressive leg edema and back pain are signs of parietal pelvic wall involvement beyond resectability. Apparent neural involvement, such as sciatic nerve impairment, is a warning sign of extrapelvic tumor involvement. However, these neural signs may be the result of previous radiotherapy or chemotherapy or both and thus must be corroborated by adequate imaging studies.

Urinary tract obstruction deserves special mention. Urinary tract obstruction is a relative contraindication for pelvic exenteration. The ureteric obstruction occurring at the ureterovesical junction is often resectable because of its central location. Upper pelvic ureteric obstruction, where the ureter travels in close proximity to the common iliac vessels and the pelvic sidewall, is more likely to be associated with unresectable disease. Table 1 shows the categorical and relative contraindications for pelvic exenteration.

Table 1
Contraindications to pelvic exenteration

Absolute	Relative
Unresectable distant metastases	Age over 70 years
Peritoneal carcinomatosis	Low pelvic ureteral obstruction
Circumferential pelvic involvement	Periosteal tumor fixation
Proximal pelvic ureteric obstruction	Moderate comorbidity
Sciatic nerve pain	Severe malnutrition
Tumor fixation with bony invasion	Nonaxial recurrence
Progressive leg edema	Short disease-free interval
Major comorbid conditions	Multiple lymph node metastases

Not withstanding the fact that a good history and physical examination can be revealing, modern imaging methods are currently relied on to determine incurability, operability, and resectability. It is worth emphasizing that a good physical examination must include local and distant lymph node regions because supraclavicular lymph node metastases, especially in locally advanced uterine cervix cancer, are not rare.

The importance of a pelvic examination under anesthesia (EUA) in the evaluation of resectability cannot be overemphasized. Although the present and other authors have shown that tumor adherence to limited portions of the pelvic bone structure is not a contraindication to resection, extensive areas of tumor fixation is, especially in the lower pelvis [6–8]. Examination of an anesthetized patient allows a careful examination of the rectum and pelvic organs, which is often limited by pain or discomfort in an awake patient. Examination under anesthesia permits a free exchange of views regarding the level and extent of tumor fixation to the pelvis as well as invasion into adjacent organs. Also, teaching of fellows, residents, and medical students may be conducted without discomfort and embarrassment to the patient. Presently, the examination can be performed using instrumentation such as rigid or flexible endoscopy and endorectal ultrasonography, which adds valuable information in an efficient manner. Table 2 shows the preoperative evaluation for pelvic exenteration.

Imaging before pelvic exenteration

The purposes of performing preoperative imaging studies are to rule out distant metastases, to establish resectability, or, in the case of suspected persistent disease, to attempt to differentiate between fibrosis and cancer recurrence. Image-directed biopsies may be ultimately required in cases in which tumor recurrence is neither clinically visible nor palpable and therefore not within the reach of a transperineal, transvaginal, or transrectal needle core biopsy. When histologic proof of recurrent malignancy is unavailable or when biopsies are negative for cancer, short-term follow-up with imaging studies may be prudent to visualize changes that in and

Table 2
Preoperative patient evaluation for pelvic exenteration

History and physical examination	Studies
Disease-free interval, stage at diagnosis	CT chest, abdomen, pelvis
Symptoms of advanced disease	Endorectal ultrasonography
Peripheral adenopathy	Pelvic MRI
Severe COPD, limited cardiac reserve	PET scanning
Nutritional state, emotional stability	Hemogram, serum chemistry
Pelvic examination under anesthesia	Liver enzymes, serum albumen
Review histology, previous radiation	Urine cultures, cystoscopy, proctoscopy
therapy and chemotherapy	(rigid), and colonoscopy
Enterostomal therapy consultation	
Pelvic reconstruction team	
Multidisciplinary oncology evaluation	
(tumor board presentations)	
Laparoscopic staging	

Abbreviations: COPD, chronic obstructive pulmonary disease; PET, positron emission tomography.

of themselves may become persuasive enough to support an exenterative procedure.

The mainstay of imaging for preoperative assessment of operability is CT scanning of the chest, abdomen, and pelvis, which can identify multiple visceral metastases that are one contraindication to exenteration for cure. A potential exception to this contraindication is patients with recurrent rectal cancer and resectable pulmonary or hepatic metastases. Common sense must prevail in this difficult decision making, because a cure is highly unlikely after the resection of an advanced primary tumor and multiple sites of metastatic disease.

A word of caution about pelvic exenteration for palliation is necessary. Although several publications attempt to justify this operation in the name of palliative care, patients who are incurable by pelvic exenteration should not, as a rule, be subjected to such a morbid procedure. The fact that exenteration can be performed with minimal mortality should not be used as an excuse to liberalize its indications. This position is based upon personal experience with the poor results of resections for recurrent pelvic cancer when gross tumor remained (R2 resections). Some important exceptions in which palliative exenteration may be advisable include young and good risk operative candidates who have limited (small tumor burden) unresectable distant disease along with symptomatic pelvic recurrence that is amenable to complete resection; patients with infected pelvic, advanced, malignant disease, which is unresponsive to percutaneous drainage or antibiotics, fistulas and obstruction that can be relieved by exenterative pelvic surgery; patients with resectable pelvic malignant disease, who have transfusion-dependent tumor bleeding and uncontrolled pain of central or visceral origin but not pelvic parietal pain.

Regardless of the reader's position this controversy, it remains the responsibility of the surgeon to educate the patient and family regarding the limited and often short-term benefits of an operation associated with a 50% complication rate and severe functional and psychologic morbidity.

In addition to CT scanning, other imaging tests are increasingly important in detecting recurrent pelvic cancer: endorectal ultrasonography (EUS), MRI, and positron emission tomography (PET). Endorectal ultrasonography has become an essential component of the pretreatment evaluation of transrectal tumor invasion, with an accuracy of over 90%. It is not as reliable as a determinant of the extent of disease in the case of recurrent pelvic cancer. When exenteration is being considered as the primary form of treatment, MRI, PET, and even pelvic EUA are more diagnostic than EUS. By the time a rectal cancer necessitates exenterative surgery, knowing the degree of transectal invasion is beyond the value of ultrasonography.

MRI for primary and recurrent pelvic cancer has been studied extensively [17]. Although it does not replace CT imaging, MRI improves the visualization of the relationship between the advancing edge of the tumor and the pelvic fascial planes and muscles. MRI is an essential component of preoperative assessment when composite resections are anticipated by virtue of pelvic wall involvement. MRI is also useful in differentiating fibrosis from tumor invasion and adds further anatomic detail to CT in up to 40% of patients. MRI has shown a sensitivity of 97% and a specificity of 98%, compared with 70% and 85% for CT.

PET scanning is a valuable adjunct in the diagnosis of local disease extent and for metastatic disease. This whole-body metabolic, rather than anatomic diagnostic, tool cannot differentiate inflammatory from neoplastic changes in the pelvis; however, it can reliably detect distant metastatic disease undiscovered by CT scanning. Also, PET has been more accurate than CT in detecting locally recurrent rectal cancer, changing clinical management in 10% to 61% of patients with recurrent rectal cancer [18,19]. In a recent publication, Staib and colleagues [18] have demonstrated that PET has an accuracy of 87% in detecting pelvic recurrence. They also showed that the positive predictive value for patients who have undergone pelvic radiotherapy within 12 months increased from 57% for CT compared with 86% for PET, although the difference did not achieve statistical significance. Combining pelvic CT and MRI imaging also is useful in predicting the likelihood of a complete resection, especially in cases with pelvic side wall tumor involvement. Among 70 patients who underwent combined CT and MRI imaging, R0 resections were performed in only 19% of cases in which imaging showed that the pelvic side wall was involved, compared with the 60% R0 resections performed in patients whose pelvic imaging showed the side wall to be free of tumor involvement [17].

From a practical and cost-effective viewpoint, imaging is best used in a progressive or sequential manner. For instance, if a CT of the abdomen and pelvis shows no evidence of distant metastasis but the EUA shows a recurrent pelvic tumor that is tethered or incompletely attached to the sacrum or pelvic sidewall in a patient having received radiation therapy, MRI is an ideal adjunct to CT because the former provides better fascial plane visualization. Furthermore, in cases in which CT-guided needle biopsy cannot confirm the presence of malignancy but malignancy is strongly suspected based on MRI, PET scanning can add a measure of diagnostic accuracy. Conversely, if a pelvic EUA demonstrates a recurrent tumor, which is freely mobile from the pelvic sidewall, and the pelvic CT confirms a visible free plane between the tumor and pelvic wall, an MRI is a superfluous examination.

The operation

Over the past 50 years, technical aspects of pelvic exenteration and its modifications have been published and have been described recently in detail [20]. It is not the intent of this article to describe the operation but to address general principles and stress the importance of good surgical judgment when technical modifications of the original procedure are desirable and feasible. For this purpose, the present senior author's 26-year experience with over 300 exenterative procedures will serve as a technical reference. As with any long-term observation, errors and successes serve as important lessons.

Staging laparoscopy for abdominopelvic malignancy before laparotomy has a definite place in the modern surgical armamentarium. The most compelling reason to use laparoscopy is because the finding of a miliary peritoneal implantation or a cytological smear showing malignant cells in peritoneal fluid or lavage, neither of which is recognizable in imaging studies, constitutes a categorical contraindication to pelvic exenteration for cure. Patients who have been so unfortunately diagnosed can be discharged immediately from the hospital, without an unnecessary abdominal incision. Although staging laparoscopy has been used primarily for upper abdominal malignancy, the use of this procedure has been reported by Köhler and colleagues [21] in patients with gynecologic malignancies who are being considered for pelvic exenteration [21]. In this study, 50% of patients were ineligible for pelvic exenteration on the basis of laparoscopic findings. It is unclear, however, if all patients underwent state-of-the-art imaging of the abdomen and pelvis before laparoscopy. The present authors advocate staging laparoscopy before exenteration for all patients in whom it is technically feasible.

Successful laparoscopic resection of pelvic organs has included radical hysterectomy, hand-assisted radical cystectomy, and abdominoperineal resection of the rectosigmoid. Pelvic lymphadenectomy through laparoscopy is common today in urologic surgery. Thus, from a technical viewpoint, there is no impediment to an oncologically sound en-bloc dissection of the entire pelvic viscera and its associated lymphatics. In fact, laparoscopy provides better visualization of deep pelvis recesses than open surgery using deep pelvic retractors. A recent publication attests to its feasibility [22]. In this anecdotal report, a 34-year-old woman with recurrent cervical carcinoma was treated with neoadjuvant chemo-radiation therapy. The progression of her disease indicated surgical salvage therapy. A subtotal pelvic exenteration with anal preservation and coloanal anastomosis was performed laparoscopically. Vulvar extraction of the specimen was accomplished, and a 5-cm abdominal incision was made to create an ileal conduit for urinary diversion. The operation lasted 9 hours.

Although there is great virtue in minimizing the size of an abdominal incision and, more important, blood loss, at present, laparoscopic pelvic exenteration for locally advanced pelvic cancer cannot be advocated as the preferred operative approach. Experience with pelvic exenteration has shown that tactile sensation plays an important role in guiding the operation, especially when portions of the pelvic viscera may be preserved. The advancing edge of the tumor can be best ascertained by palpation of the viscera as dissection progresses. Although the gross margin required for an R0 resection is generally 2 cm, the failure to anticipate the required tissue resection margins can make a potentially curative resection into a palliative one.

The four main types of pelvic exenteration are anterior, posterior, supralevator, and total exenteration. The first two types are used almost exclusively in women with recurrent cervical or rectal cancer, owing to the presence of the internal genitalia as a barrier to tumor extension. For women with cervical cancer involving the anterior vaginal wall and vesico-vaginal septum, an anterior exenteration often suffices, whereas a posterior exenteration for recurrent low rectal cancer usually includes an extended abdominoperineal resection with en-bloc resection of uterus, adnexa, and posterior vaginal wall, thus preserving the bladder. In men, an axial or central pelvic recurrence of rectal cancer generally involves the periprostatic or vesical area, and a partial pelvic exenteration often is not feasible. It is permissible to attempt bladder preservation in selected cases of limited posterior involvement of the urinary tract.

The present authors previously published a detailed description of patient positioning and other preparatory maneuvers for pelvic exenteration, with an emphasis on details not generally addressed in publications on this subject [20]. For instance, opening the para-aortic retroperitoneal space is critical in determining resectability for cure, especially for recurrent cervical and low rectal carcinomas in the absence of extrapelvic, intraperitoneal tumor spread. Tumor fixation within the pelvis cannot be ascertained without opening the pelvic peritoneum from the promontory of the sacrum along the brim of the pelvis to the bladder on the side where the tumor is closest to the pelvic side wall. Also, sharp mobilization of the posterior part of the rectum down to the sacrorectal ligament and the bladder anterolaterally permits the surgeon to assess mobility and the lateral extent of the tumor. These maneuvers often determine whether complete tumor excision is possible well before transection of the ureters, colon, and visceral blood supply.

Following the anterior and posterior avascular dissection and having determined the type of resection required, the sacrorectal ligament is sharply divided to permit a complete resection of the mesorectum. The lateral pelvic dissection is initiated by mobilizing the ureter medially, and the parietal layer of the endopelvic fascia is divided medial to the genitofemoral nerve. It is important to preserve this nerve and the obturator nerve because there are no lymph nodes lateral to these structures, which lie over the psoas and obturator muscles, respectively. The vascular sheath of the internal iliac vessels is dissected cleanly to ligate and divide visceral vessels at their origin, rather than as soft tissue pedicles, which leaves lymphoareolar tissue behind. There is no need to ligate the main internal iliac vessels because it unnecessarily sacrifices parietal pelvic blood supply. The dissection proceeds down to the levator muscle, which is best divided from the perineum. Because the dissection is identical on both sides, this operation provides an excellent opportunity to demonstrate the dissection by the senior member of the surgical team performing the side closest to the tumor and to assist a senior trainee or junior faculty member on the other side. The rest of the lateral pelvic dissection includes identifying and preserving the sacral plexus. This nerve plexus is composed of the fourth and fifth lumbar roots and is situated dorsally and laterally from the obturator nerve. The levator ani muscle originates from the fascia of the obturator internus muscle. Once this muscle is demonstrated circumferentially, the rectum is mobilized to the coccyx, the bladder is mobilized to the periurethral region, and the perineal dissection can begin.

In men, the perineal incision is made from the base of the scrotum, around the sutured anus, to the tip of the coccyx. In women, the labia majora are sutured in line with the anus, thus obliterating the entire perineum to avoid contamination from vaginal tumor involvement, and the incision is made lateral to the vulva, around the sutured anus to the tip of the coccyx. Exceptions to the extent of these incisions can be made if the vulva and vagina are completely uninvolved by tumor and a supralevator exenteration is anticipated. In men, the proximal end of the penile urethra is suture ligated and divided. For transitional urothelial carcinomas, the entire penile urethra can be dissected through a ventral penile incision as prophylaxis against urethral cancer. The entire contents of the ischiorectal space is dissected until the urogenital diaphragm is exposed. It is preferable to first enter the pelvic space posteriorly and then laterally, leaving the retropubic dissection as the last maneuver before extracting the specimen. After complete hemostasis is achieved, it is imperative that the surgeon orient the specimen in the presence of the pathologist and that the surgical resection margins are inked for histologic study.

Pelvic reconstruction has been associated with a significant reduction of morbidity from this radical procedure [23]. When the greater omentum is of generous size, an omental flap can fill the lower pelvis. Other means of pelvic reconstruction have been reported using various myocutaneous flaps [24]. A description of reconstructive techniques is beyond the scope of this article, but the importance of reconstruction cannot be minimized. Similarly, urinary diversion has evolved since Bricker's original description [3]. Although the ileal conduit remains the present authors' preferred approach for urinary diversion, continent conduits and neobladder reconstructions have come of age and are recommended when they are performed by surgeons who have experience with these elaborate procedures.

Morbidity and mortality of pelvic exenteration

As with any major oncologic procedure, pelvic exenteration has evolved and been made safer by a number of improvements in the care of the surgical patient. Bricker and other pioneers, faced with the challenges of primitive anesthesia and intraoperative monitoring and inherent difficulties with transfusion and other volume replacement techniques, resorted to speed in surgical performance to minimize operating time and blood loss, which at times was massive. The resection portion of pelvic exenteration, which today takes an average of 3 hours, often was performed by Bricker in approximately 90 minutes, 1 hour in the abdomen and 30 minutes in the perineal portion. Mortality from hypovolemia and probable myocardial injury was not uncommon, but the majority of operative mortality from total pelvic exenteration did not occur predominantly intraoperatively or in the early postoperative period. Most of the 30-day mortality, as high as 20% in the 1950s, was caused by postoperative septic complications and the impact of radiation enteritis on small intestinal loops caught in the empty and denuded pelvic cavity, resulting in frequent episodes of intestinal obstruction and fistulas. In the era before parenteral nutrition, these complications demanded prompt operative intervention, adding to the morbidity of the initial operation.

As noted in the present authors' 1999 review on this subject, most of the literature implies that morbidity from this procedure is only an immediate postoperative phenomenon [20]. A report of a 50-year institutional experience with this procedure attests to the fact that morbidity must be measured on a long-term basis [5]. The 30-day morbidity rate among 232 patients after pelvic exenteration, treated between 1950 and 1990, was 45%. However, 75 of 191 (39%) patients discharged from the hospital developed one or more complications after 30 days, attributable directly to the operation. To our knowledge, this is the only report of a reliably conducted long-term morbidity monitoring study after exenteration.

The contemporary experience with exenterative pelvic surgery suggests that morbidity from this operation remains high, whereas operative mortality has decreased to less than 5%. Table 3 shows morbidity, mortality, and survival rates for pelvic exenteration in selected series in patients who underwent operations within the last 15 years [25–31]. In a recent publication of the authors' experience with composite pelvic exenteration, the operative mortality was 0%, but the morbidity rate was 67% [6]. Among 26 complications occurring in 13 patients, more than 50% were of septic origin, but intestinal fistulas, intestinal obstruction, and sacral wound dehiscence contributed significantly to surgical morbidity rates. Generally, the currently low mortality rates from this type of cancer surgery are caused by our ability to effectively manage complications while preserving the nutritional state of these patients. Jejunostomy feeding is highly desirable after pelvic exenteration. Modern imaging permits nonoperative management of intra-abdominal sepsis, decreasing reoperation rates, which contributed to increased mortality in previous decades.

Contemporary survival results after pelvic exenteration

The multidisciplinary modern day treatment of advanced pelvic malignancy requires that the long-term results of exenterative surgery be

Table 3
Selected contemporary series of pelvic exenterations for rectal cancer

Study	Year	N	Morbidity (%)	Mortality (%)	5-y survival (recurrent) (%)	5-y survival (primary) (%)	Overall survival (%)
Law et al [31]	2000	24	54	0	0	64	44
Kecmanovic et al [9]	2003	28	43	10	17	32	N/A
Chen and Sheen-Chen [10]	2001	50	37	2	—	49	49
Kakuda et al [27]	2003	22	68	6	Median survival/20 months	—	—
Jimenez et al [25]	2003	55	78	5	28	77	40
Oliveira et al [29]	2004	44	62	15	N/A	N/A	41
Gonzalez et al [30]	2003[c]	45	56	4	32	31	31
Ike et al [16]	2003[a]	71	66	4	—	54	54
Ike et al [28]	2003[b]	45	77	13	14	—	14
Wiig et al [11]	2002	47	38	4	18	36	28
Yamada et al [26]	2002	64	50	2	23	60	32
Vitelli et al [12]	2003	26	46	11	N/A	N/A	58
Lopez and Luna-Pérez [6]	2004[d]	19	67	0	44	—	44

Abbreviation: N/A, not applicable.
[a] Total pelvic exenteration for primary rectal cancer.
[b] Total pelvic exenteration for recurrent rectal cancer.
[c] Transsacral exenteration.
[d] Composite exenteration.

examined on the basis of recent experience [25]. Neoadjuvant chemo-radiation therapy, used as early as 1974 for the treatment of patients with anal squamous cell carcinoma, generally was not used to treat patients with other pelvic cancers until the late 1980s. Experience with exenteration following neoadjuvant therapy was anecdotal before 1990. Several recent publications have contributed to increasing knowledge of the natural history of pelvic cancers treated with combined modality [25,27–31]. There has long been evidence that preoperative therapy converts to resectable some rectosigmoid carcinomas that were originally deemed unresectable, usually because of pelvic or sacral fixation. With the evident down-staging effect of neoadjuvant therapy, patients with locally advanced pelvic malignancy should be considered for preoperative treatment. However, in patients with primary locally advanced rectal cancer that is centrally located within the pelvis and with vaginal or bladder penetration, treatment will not change the magnitude of the operation. Admittedly, this group of patients represents a minority because most patients who are candidates for exenterative surgery have recurrent neoplasms after treatment with surgery, radiation, or chemotherapy alone or in combination. All patients with rectal cancer treated with total or partial pelvic exenteration for primary rectal cancer benefit from adjuvant postoperative therapy because, by definition, they have T4 and possibly N+ tumors. Promising results of intraoperative high-dose pelvic irradiation with brachytherapy suggests that the local control rate may be further enhanced in patients undergoing pelvic exenteration, especially for nonaxial recurrences [32].

Even the current literature on results of pelvic exenteration is marred by the heterogeneity of the patient population. Moreover, information on factors known to affect recurrence and survival rates is often missing. For instance, most reports do not provide information on lymph node status, microscopically examined surgical resection margins, analyses of recurrence, and survival results for surgery performed for primary or recurrent disease, whether or not patients were treated with pre- or postoperative adjuvant therapy, and what such therapy entailed. Even when adjuvant therapy has been used, it frequently is unknown whether external beam alone or in conjunction with brachytherapy was administered. Information on chemo-therapy is missing from most reports, and in those that have some infor-mation, it is unclear whether it was administered by continuous infusion or was given concurrently with pelvic irradiation.

With the above caveats, a review of selected, recent reports may provide an understanding of morbidity and survival results from pelvic exenteration. Table 3 shows a summary of selected contemporary series of exenterations for rectal cancer. Although the 13 series published from 2000 to 2003 reported an average of 43 patients each, a total of 540 patients is included in this summary, and some general conclusions can be reached.

Morbidity and mortality are universally being reported. Some series report all morbidities, whereas others report only major morbidity. Because "major" morbidity is difficult to define, it is fair to state that the average reported morbidity rate of 50% is no different from the 50-year institutional experience reported by the present authors [5]. Pelvic exenteration is morbid in physical as well as psychologic terms. Psychologic morbidity is almost never measured. The nature of the complications in these series is listed in Table 4. They are no different from those reported in previous decades [5,21]. Operative morbidity rarely translates into operative mortality because of the sophisticated nature of current perioperative care. Operative mortality has declined over time, but the authors believe that deaths attributed to pelvic exenteration have reached a level over the last decade owing, in part, to unpredictable serious morbidity such as myocardial infarction and to the inclusion of older patients as candidates for this radical operation. Even when the exenteration is extended to include bony portions of the pelvis, the so-called composite pelvic exenteration, morbidity remained unchanged for 15 years, whereas mortality was 0% during the same period.

Recurrence and survival results, especially disease-specific survival, also are often missing from published reports. In Table 3, an attempt has been made to identify the survival results of exenteration performed for primary rectal cancer and for recurrent rectal cancer. Few reports address the type of oncologic resection performed, whether surgical resection margins were histologically tumor-free (R0 resection), margins were microscopically involved (R1), or there was residual gross tumor (R2). It is likely that when published reports separate results for curative versus palliative procedures, the results will correlate to R0, R1, and R2 resections, respectively. Table 5 shows the results of four recent series reporting survival by resection type. The average 5-year overall survival of 35% for R0 resection shown is not significantly different from the overall survival of 38%

Table 4
Complications of pelvic exenteration for rectal cancer

Complication	Rate range (%)
Wound infection	8–49
Abscess (abdominal, pelvic)	9–38
Fistula (enteral, vaginal, perineal)	3–18
Intestinal obstruction	2–33
Urinary complication	2–20
Anastomotic leaks	2–23
Cardiopulmonary	2–18
Perineal wound dehiscence	4–40
Postoperative bleeding	2–11
Deep vein thrombosis	3–8
Pulmonary embolism	4–5
Stomal hernia	3–5
Sepsis	2–10
Other	3–10

2000–2003 data from Refs. [6,9–12,16,25–31].

Table 5
Complete R0 resection and survival in patients treated by pelvic exenteration

Study	Year	N	R0 survival (%)	R1–R2 survival (%)
Oliviera et al [29]	2004	96	40-month median	21-month median
Ike et al [16]	2003	45	31 at 5-y	7 R0 and 0 R2
Wiig et al [11]	2002	47	36	18
Yamada et al [26]	2002	64	32	0

as shown in Table 3 for all patients treated for "cure." Similarly, the dismal 5% average 5-year survival rate for patients undergoing R1 or R2 resection is comparable to the reported 5-year survival of nearly 0% for palliative exenterations. In another recent confirmatory article, Shoup and colleagues [33] reported more than twice the survival rates for patients undergoing an R0 resection compared with those undergoing an R1 or R2 resection.

The present authors' experience and review of the literature support the use of pelvic exenteration for recurrent rectal cancer. However, there is a paucity of literature regarding the impact on survival, if any, of true recurrence (defined as following a period of clinical disease-free survival) when compared with persistent disease after nonsurgical treatment or residual disease following an incomplete resection of a primary tumor. Often, these terms are used interchangeably in the literature, to the detriment of data interpretation. We agree with the importance of defining pelvic regions of recurrent disease when planning surgical therapy or interpreting factors affecting outcome, as has been reported by Moore and colleagues [17]. In their experience, when pelvic sidewall involvement was suspected clinically or by CT and MRI, R0 resection was possible in less than 20% of patients, compared with an R0 resection rate of 60% when these findings were absent.

The 5-year survival rates for recurrent rectal cancer treated by pelvic exenteration range from 0% to 32%. The average for the seven series reporting separate survival for recurrent rectal cancer is 18% (see Table 3). This salvage rate is probably the result of a higher percentage of R1 and R2 resections in this group of patients, most of whom had undergone previous surgical resection of a rectosigmoid primary. Jimenez and associates [25] have shown that survival after pelvic exenteration was significantly better in patients who did not undergo abdominoperineal resection, compared with those who did. As the present authors have consistently taught to surgical residents, recurrences present a challenge that is directly proportional to the extent of the previous pelvic dissection. The logical extension of this thinking is that when surgeons are confronted with a technical challenge beyond their capabilities, it is in the best interest of the patient's future treatment to avoid pelvic visceral resections that are unlikely to achieve an R0 resection. Sound clinical judgment dictates that the best course of action under these circumstances is to close the abdomen and refer the patient to a center with surgical and multidisciplinary expertise in this field.

Patterns of failure after pelvic exenteration remain unchanged over the last 2 decades. It is hoped that the future results of exenterated patients who have received concurrent chemotherapy and whole pelvic irradiation, either pre- or postoperatively, will reflect an improved local control rate after aggressive pelvic surgery. Recent data suggest that local failures after pelvic exenteration are still at an average of 20% [25]. When tumor extent requires a composite pelvic exenteration, the recurrence rates increase to approximately 30%, as reported by Gonzalez and associates [6], almost identical to the recurrence rate in our reported series.

Factors determining complete (R0) resectability for recurrent rectal cancer are almost intuitive to surgeons experienced in pelvic cancer surgery, but they have been carefully studied. Factors include male gender, previous abdominoperineal resection, carcinoembryonic antigen-positive tumors, high p53 proto-oncogene expression, lymphovascular tumor invasion, advanced patient age at the time of diagnosis, advanced stage of the primary tumor, hydronephrosis and tumor proximity to the pelvic sidewall, and low surgical volume [34]. All of the above factors can be summarized as follows: Unfavorable tumor biology, nonaxial tumor recurrence, poor patient selection, previous extensive surgery, and surgical inexperience are all unfavorable prognostic indicators.

In summary, pelvic exenteration remains a challenging procedure with significant morbidity. A multidisciplinary approach to treatment evaluation of recurrent pelvic malignancy is paramount to success. This operation must be performed in centers with dedicated expertise, although there are reports of successes in smaller institutions where trained personnel are available. The operation has evolved along with imaging, perioperative care, and adjuvant therapy. It has retained its place in the armamentarium of surgeons with interest in pelvic cancer surgery. Bricker said it well in his last contribution to the surgical literature: "Ordinarily, after 40 years, a new operation will have been discarded or so modified and improved that its origin becomes unrecognizable and is forgotten. The fact that there is still a place for the comparatively simple concept behind the early operation—and the knowledge that it still serves a useful purpose—is a great boost to my ego."

References

[1] Brunschwig A. Complete excision of pelvic viscera for advanced carcinoma: a one-stage abdominoperineal operation with end colostomy and bilateral ureteral implantation into the colon above the colostomy. Cancer 1948;1:177–83.

[2] Spratt JS, Watson FR, Pratt JL. Characteristics of variants of colorectal carcinoma that do not metastasize to lymph nodes. Dis Colon Rectum 1970;13:243–6.

[3] Bricker EM. Bladder substitution after pelvic evisceration. Surg Clin North Am 1950;30: 1511–21.

[4] Spratt JS, Butcher HR, Bricker EM. Exenterative surgery of the pelvis. Philadelphia: WB Saunders; 1973.

[5] Lopez MJ, Standiford SB, Skibba JL. Total pelvic exenteration: a 50-year experience at the Ellis Fischel Cancer Center. Arch Surg 1994;129:390–6.

[6] Lopez MJ, Luna-Pérez P. Composite pelvic exenteration: is it worthwhile? Ann Surg Oncol 2003;11(1):27–33.

[7] Wanebo HJ, Gaker DL, Whitehill R, et al. Pelvic recurrence of rectal cancer. Ann Surg 1987; 205:482–94.

[8] Yamada K, Ishizawa T, Kiyoshi N, et al. Pelvic exenteration and sacral resection for locally advanced primary and recurrent rectal cancer. Dis Colon Rectum 2002;45(8):1078–84.

[9] Kecmanovic DM, Pavlov MJ, Kovacevic PA, et al. Management of advanced pelvic cancer by exenteration. Eur J Surg Oncol 2003;29:743–6.

[10] Chen HS, Sheen-Chen SM. Total pelvic exenteration for primary local advanced colorectal cancer. World J Surg 2001;25:1546–9.

[11] Wiig JN, Poulsen JP, Larsen S, et al. Total pelvic exenteration with preoperative irradiation for advanced primary and recurrent rectal cancer. Eur J Surg 2002;168:42–8.

[12] Vitelli CE, Crenca F, Fortunato L, et al. Pelvic exenterative procedures for locally advanced or recurrent colorectal carcinoma in a community hospital. Tech Coloproctol 2003;7: 159–63.

[13] Spratt JS, Spjut HJ. Prevalence and prognosis of individual clinical and pathologic variables associated with colorectal carcinoma. Cancer 1967;20:1976–85.

[14] Gall FP, Hermanek P. Change and current status of surgical treatment of colorectal cancer: report of experience of the Erlangen Surgical University Clinic. Chirurg 1992;63(4): 227–34.

[15] Lopez MJ, Kraybill WG, Downey R, et al. Exenterative surgery for locally advanced rectosigmoid cancers: is it worthwhile? Surgery 1987;102:644–51.

[16] Ike H, Shimada H, Yamaguchi S, et al. Outcome of total pelvic exenteration for primary rectal cancer. Dis Colon Rectum 2003;46(4):474–80.

[17] Moore HG, Shoup M, Riedel E, et al. Colorectal cancer pelvic recurrences: determinants of resectability. Dis Colon Rectum 2004;47(10):1599–606.

[18] Staib L, Schirrmeister H, Reske SN, et al. Is ^{18}F-fluorodeoxyglucose positron emission tomography in recurrent colorectal cancer a contribution to surgical decision making? Am J Surg 2000;180:1–5.

[19] Whiteford MH, Whiteford HM, Yee LF, et al. Usefulness of FDG-PET scan in the assessment of suspected metastatic or recurrent adenocarcinoma of the colon and rectum. Dis Colon Rectum 2000;43(6):759–70.

[20] Lopez MJ, Spratt JS. Exenterative pelvic surgery. J Surg Oncol 1999;72:102–14.

[21] Köhler C, Tozzi R, Possover M, et al. Explorative laparoscopy prior to exenterative surgery. Gynecol Oncol 2002;86:311–5.

[22] Pomel C, Rouzier R, Pocard M, et al. Laparoscopic total pelvic exenteration for cervical cancer relapse. Gynecol Oncol 2003;91:616–8.

[23] Jurado M, Bazán A, Elejabeitia J, et al. Primary vaginal and pelvic floor reconstruction at the time of pelvic exenteration: a study of morbidity. Gynecol Oncol 2000;77:293–7.

[24] Tobin GR. Pelvic, vaginal, and perineal reconstruction in radical pelvic surgery. Surg Oncol Clin N Am 1994;3(2):397–413.

[25] Jimenez RE, Shoup M, Cohen AM, et al. Contemporary outcomes of total pelvic exenteration in the treatment of colorectal cancer. Dis Colon Rectum 2003;46(12):1619–25.

[26] Yamada K, Ishizawa T, Niwa K, et al. Pelvic exenteration and sacral resection for locally advanced primary and recurrent rectal cancer. Dis Colon Rectum 2002;45:1078–84.

[27] Kakuda JT, Lamont JP, Chu DZJ, et al. The role of pelvic exenteration in the management of recurrent rectal cancer. Am J Surg 2003;186:660–4.

[28] Ike H, Shimada H, Ohki S, et al. Outcome of total pelvic exenteration for locally recurrent rectal cancer. Hepato-gastroenterology 2003;50:700–3.

[29] Oliveira Poletto AH, Lopes A, Carvalho AL, et al. Pelvic exenteration and sphincter preservation: an analysis of 96 cases. J Surg Oncol 2004;86:122–7.

[30] Gonzalez RJ, McCarter MD, McDermott T, et al. Transsacral exenteration of fixed primary and recurrent anorectal cancer. Am J Surg 2003;186:670–4.
[31] Law WK, Chu KW, Choi HK. Total pelvic exenteration for locally advanced rectal cancer. J Am Coll Surg 2000;190(1):78–83.
[32] Alektiar KM, Zelefsky MJ, Paty PB, et al. High-dose rate intraoperative brachytherapy for recurrent colorectal cancer. Int J Radiat Oncol Biol Phys 2000;48:219–26.
[33] Shoup M, Guillem JG, Alektiar KM, et al. Predictors of survival in recurrent rectal cancer after resection and intraoperative radiotherapy. Dis Colon Rectum 2002;45(5):585–92.
[34] Begg CB, Cramer LD, Hoskins WJ, et al. Impact of Hospital Volume on Operative Mortality for Major Cancer Surgery. JAMA 1998;280:1747–51.

ELSEVIER
SAUNDERS

Surg Oncol Clin N Am
14 (2005) 607–631

SURGICAL
ONCOLOGY CLINICS
OF NORTH AMERICA

Radical Gynecologic Surgery for Cancer

Sarah H. Hughes, MD[a,b], Michael A. Steller, MD[a,b,*]

[a]Division of Gynecologic Oncology, Caritas St. Elizabeth's Medical Center
of Boston, 736 Cambridge Street, Boston, MA 02135-2997, USA
[b]Tufts University School of Medicine, 136 Harrison Avenue, Boston,
MA 02111, USA

Radical pelvic surgery continues to figure prominently in the clinical management of gynecologic malignancies. The history of radical gynecologic cancer surgery extends back to the late 1800s, before the development of adequate anesthesia, aseptic technique, or antibiotics. Throughout the 1900s many dedicated gynecologic surgeons studied their procedures and outcomes, forming the basis for current therapies in gynecology oncology. This article describes a short history and current radical surgical treatments for cervical, ovarian, endometrial, and vulvar cancers.

Cervical cancer

Cervical cancer is the second most common cancer among women worldwide, with approximately 450,000 new cases diagnosed each year, and nearly 200,000 deaths annually are attributable to this disease [1]. Although the widespread use of Papanicolaou smears has resulted in a 70% decline in the mortality from cervical cancer in the United States during the past 50 years [2], cervical cancer remains a leading cause of cancer-related death in women in developing countries. In developed countries, successful screening has lowered the incidence of cervical cancer, at an estimated cost of nearly $6 billion annually in the United States alone [3].

During the past quarter century, a causal link between the human papillomavirus (HPV) and a variety of anogenital cancers has been firmly established. Genital HPV infections are estimated to have the highest incidence of any sexually transmitted disease in the United States [4]. Extensive epidemiologic data has strongly associated HPV with a spectrum of anogenital neoplasms, including condylomata (genital warts), cervical

---

* Corresponding author. Division of Gynecologic Oncology, Caritas St. Elizabeth's Medical Center of Boston, 736 Cambridge Street, Boston, MA 02135-2997.

  E-mail address: Michael_Steller@cchcs.org (M.A. Steller).

1055-3207/05/$ - see front matter © 2005 Elsevier Inc. All rights reserved.
doi:10.1016/j.soc.2005.04.004   *surgonc.theclinics.com*

dysplasia, and cervical carcinoma. HPV DNA is detected in more than 99% of all tumors of the uterine cervix [5].

Despite the impressive advances in our understanding of the natural history, epidemiology, virology, and immunology associated with cervical cancer, it remains a clinically challenging disease for which therapy often involves radical pelvic surgery. Because cervical cancer is most prevalent in settings where access to modern medical technology is often limited, this disease continues to be staged by physical examination and selected radiographic studies, rather than surgical criteria. Squamous cell carcinoma accounts for approximately 85% of all cervical malignancies, while adeno-carcinoma comprises almost all of the remaining cases. Clincally, these two histologic varieties of cervical cancer are treated similarly, with no appreciable difference in outcome. In current practice, therapy is determined by stage, and can include surgery, radiation therapy, as well as sensitizing chemotherapy used in conjunction with radiation. Therapy is aimed at removing the primary tumor and addressing routes of metastasis.

History

The radical hysterectomy is the most common surgical procedure for cervical cancer. Although Ernst Wertheim is most famous for the development of the radical hysterectomy, a great deal of work was done before him. The origins of the surgical approach to this disease began in the eighteenth century, when surgical removal was suggested by Osiander and Wresberg [6]. As reported by Zweifel, in 1821 Sauter performed the first vaginal hysterectomy for cervical cancer [7]. At that time, the understanding of aseptic technique, combined with limited anesthetic methods and no antibiotics, greatly limited successful outcomes. In 1878, the abdominal hysterectomy began with W.A. Freund, who performed an abdominal surgery consisting of extirpation, followed by three mass ligatures on each side. The surgical mortality was near 32% [8]. One of Freund's assistants, Linkenheld, found that Freund's patients usually had a recurrence within 2.5 years [9]. He suggested a more radical surgery and, in 1881, Freund performed a hysterectomy with removal of the parametria. Around the same time other surgeons, like Mackenrodt, in1894, began to favor parametrial excision. Clark (while a resident at Johns Hopkins in the 1890s) favored removing the broad ligament to the lateral pelvic wall while also removing the upper vagina [9]. In Vienna, in 1898, Ernst Wertheim performed the first radical hysterectomy and partial lymphadenectomy for cervical cancer. His results, published in 1911, showed a 10% operative mortality compared to 50% in earlier reports [10]. In the early 1900s, attempts at a vaginal approach were made once again. Schauta, of Vienna, performed an extensive vaginal operation with a mortality rate of 10% and a 5-year survival of 40%. Since Wertheim's time several surgeons have modified the radical hysterectomy. At the turn of the century (1905) Burnet extended the parametrial excision, as did Joe Meigs, who went to Vienna in the 1930s to learn the Wertheim operation. Meigs helped to revitalize the surgical approach to cervical cancer in the last century, publishing his operative treatment in 1944 [11].

The incorporation of lymphadenectomy came from experience with axillary lymph node dissection in breast cancer. Anatomic studies in the 1800s by Cruveilhier in 1834 and Wagner in 1858 found positive nodes in patients who died from cervical cancer [12,13]. In addition, it was found that the parametria contained abnormal lymph nodes before they were palpably abnormal. Several surgeons pioneered lymphadenectomy at the early part of the twentieth century [14,15]. Meigs reintroduced lymphadenectomy in the United States in the 1940s as part of the radical surgical treatment of cervical cancer [11]. In 1967, the International Federation of Gynecology and Obstetrics (FIGO) declared the standard for radical lymphadenectomy would encompass the removal of at least 20 lymph nodes.

Radiation therapy also has an important and well-established role in the management of cervical cancer. In 1898, Madam Marie Curie discovered radium, and in the early 1902 it was found that patients had lower mortality rates and improved survival when treated with radiation compared to surgery. For several decades radiation was the standard of care for cervical cancer, with lower mortality than surgical approaches. As data accrued, it was discovered that survival was only 40%. This drove an increase in radiation dosages, and then the complication rate increased. However, in 1941, Victor Bonney [16] presented a series of 500 cervical cancer patients who were treated with surgery. His series had an operative mortality of 14% and 5-year survival rate of 42%. At the same time that the complications of radiation therapy were starting to be appreciated, Bonney illustrated that surgical success was comparable to radiation. This began the trend toward operative management of early stage cervical cancer.

A classification schema for extended hysterectomy was proposed by Piver and Rutledge in 1974, and is divided into five types of surgery [17]. Type I consists of a simple extrafascial hysterectomy. Type II is a modified radical hysterectomy where the ureters are dissected to the paracervical tunnel, the cardinal ligaments are resected at the level of the ureter, and the uterosacral ligaments are partially resected (Figs. 1 and 2). Type III is performed like a type II, with the addition of bilateral lymphadeneactomy. Type IV is an extended radical hysterectomy where the superior vesical artery is sacrificed and more of the vaginal cuff is removed. Last, the Type V radical hysterectomy includes removal of the distal ureter or bladder; this extended hysterectomy is tantamount to an anterior pelvic exenteration.

Pelvic exenteration also has a place in the treatment of cervical cancer, and is performed for several indications: stage IV disease, central recurrence of disease, and palliation of complications from radiation therapy such as fistulae. This extremely radical procedure is covered in more detail in articles by Lopez and Garrett and colleagues elsewhere in this issue. Briefly, it

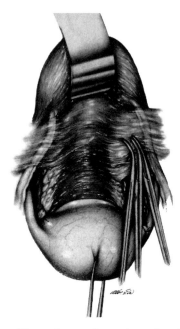

Fig. 1. Type II hysterectomy: The uterine vessels are clamped medial to the ureters, which are dissected to the paracervical tunnel. The medial third of the cardinal ligament is removed. (*From* Rock JA, Thomspon JD, editors. TeLinde's operative gynecology, 8th edition. Philadelphia: Lippincott, Williams & Wilkins; 1997; with permission.)

includes a radical hysterectomy and pelvic lymphadenectomy. An anterior pelvic exenteration consists of removing the bladder, whereas an posterior pelvic exenteration involves removal of the rectum. A total pelvic exenteration combines the two. The perineal phase of an exenteration involves removal of the vagina and anus. The operative mortality ranges from 2% to 13.5%, and the 5-year survival is between 25% and 61% [18].

Therapeutic considerations

Current therapy is determined by clinical stage, and was outlined in the National Institutes of Health Consensus Statement published in 1996 [19] (Table 1). Microinvasive cancers (stage IA1) can be treated with either cone biopsy or simple hysterectomy. The diagnosis of state IA1 must be made by cone biopsy, and not by cervical punch biopsy alone. The current surgical approach is based on the understanding that lymph node involvement is related to the depth of tumor invasion: the greater the depth, the greater the risk of invasion. With a stage IA1 tumor, the risk of lymph node involvement is <1%; therefore, treatment usually requires less extensive surgery. During the past decade, it has been recognized that patients with microinvasive squamous cell carcinomas of the cervix and evidence of lymphatic vascular space invasion have a substantially increased risk of

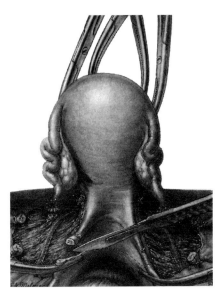

Fig. 2. Partial resection of cardinal ligament. (*From* Rock JA, Thomspon JD, editors. TeLinde's operative gynecology. 8th edition. Philadelphia: Lippincott, Williams & Wilkins, 1997; with permission.)

regional lymph node metastases, leading some to recommend more extensive surgery when this clinical entity is identified [20]. If a patient is found to have greater than stage IA1 disease after a simple hysterectomy is performed, she can be treated with either radiation therapy after surgery, or a subsequent surgery involving radical parametrectomy and pelvic lymphadenectomy.

Because the depth of invasion with stage IA2 cervical cancer increases the risk of lymph node metastasis, a radical or modified radical hysterectomy is necessary. If a patient's comorbidities preclude surgery, she may be treated with primary radiation therapy. Patients with stages IB and IIA cancer can be treated with either radical hysterectomy and pelvic lymphadenectomy or radiation therapy. Extensive clinical data demonstrate that therapeutic success is equivalent with either radical surgery or radiation therapy, although the potential toxicities differ considerably. Radical hysterectomy can result in urologic complications, such as injury to the ureters, and dysfunction of the bladder. Lymphadenectomy may result in direct vascular injury, as well as lymphatic complications such as lymphocysts and lymphedema. Radiation therapy may injure the area surrounding the cervix and parametria, primarily affecting the vagina, bladder, intestines, and rectum. The vagina often becomes narrowed, causing dyspareunia with sexual intercourse. The bowel, which is more vulnerable to radiation injury than the bladder, may develop proctosigmoiditis, and this may progress to ulcerations and strictures. Any bowel present in the pelvis is vulnerable to

Table 1
Cervical cancer FIGO staging

0	Carcinoma in situ
1	Cervical carcinoma confined to uterus (extension to corpus should be disregarded)
IA	Invasive carcinoma diagnosed only by microscopy. Stromal invasion with a maximum depth of 5.0 mm measured from the based of the epithelium and a horizontal spread of 7.0 mm or less. Vascular space involvement, venous or lymphatic, does not affect classification.
IA1	Measured stromal invasion of 3.0 mm or less in depth and 7.0 mm or less in horizontal spread.
IA2	Measured stromal invasion more than 3.0 mm and not more than 5.0 mm with a horizontal spread of 7.0 mm or less.
IB	Clinically visible lesion confined to the cervix or microscopic lesion greater than IA2
IB1	Clinically visible lesion 4.0 cm or less in greatest dimension
IB2	Clinically visible lesion more than 4.0 cm in greatest diameter
II	Cervical carcinoma invades beyond uterus but not to pelvic wall or to lower third of vagina.
IIA	Tumor without parametrial involvement
IIB	Tumor with parametrial involvement
III	Tumor extends to pelvic wall and/or involves lower third of vagina, and/or causes hydronephrosis or nonfunctioning kidney
IIIA	Tumor involves lower third of vagina, no extension to pelvic wall
IIIB	Tumor extends to pelvic wall and/or causes hydronephrosis or nonfunctioning kidney
IVA	Tumor invades mucosa of bladder or rectum, and/or extends beyond true pelvis

the effects of radiation, potentially, forming enterovaginal or enterocutaneaous fistulas. Bladder injuries can occur, with fistulas usually occurring as a delayed radiation induced complication.

Until the mid 1990s, combined surgical and radiation therapy was commonly used to treat cervical cancer. This was first described by Stallworth, a disciple of Booney, who used pretreatment radiation therapy followed by extensive parametrial dissection and lymph node dissection 4 to 6 weeks later [6]. The surgical goal was to remove the uterine isthmus and myometrium, after radiation treated the parametria, upper vagina, and pelvic nodes. This approach was primarily used for bulky or barrel shaped disease. This fell out of favor when it was discovered that it only increased cost and patient morbidity. Currently patients with stage IIB and greater disease usually are treated with external beam radiation and brachytherapy, with or without sensitizing chemotherapy.

In 1999, the National Cancer Institute published an alert stating that patients with cervical cancer requiring treatment with radiation should be offered concurrent chemotherapy [21]. This was based on data from five randomized clinical trials with a total of 1894 patients showing improved outcome for treatment with chemoradiotherapy compared with standard radiation therapy alone [22–26]. A 2003 review by Green and colleagues [27] supports combining chemotherapy with radiation therapy for cervical cancer.

Efforts during the past 15 years have been directed at less radical surgery that maintains good outcomes and preserves fertility. Dargent and colleagues [28] were the first to describe a radical vaginal trachelectomy combined with a laparoscopic pelvic lymphadenectomy to treat early-stage invasive cervical cancer. In 2000, the group presented their results with 47 patients operated on between 1987 and 1996. There were five cases of stage IA1, 14 cases of stage IA2, 25 cases of stage IB, and 3 cases of stage IIB cervical cancer. The mean follow-up was 52 months, with two recurrences and one patient death from disease progression. This procedure requires rigorous selection criteria, including FIGO stages IA2–IB, lesion <2 cm, limited endocervical involvement at colposcopy, no evidence of lymph node metastasis, and absence of vascular space invasion [29]. At the time of surgery, a laparoscopic pelvic lymphadenectomy is performed, and the lymph nodes are sent for frozen section [30–32]. Only if the nodes are negative is a radical vaginal trachelectomy performed. If the tumor extends to the margins, a radical vaginal hysterectomy in the Schauta method is performed. In 2004, Kolioppoulos and colleagues [29] reviewed the literature on radical vaginal trachelectomy, consisting mostly of case–control studies comparing radical vaginal trachelectomy with radical abdominal hysterectomy, and found that the recurrence rates ranged from 0% to 8%. This is comparable to the overall recurrence rates for radical abdominal hysterectomy. Although there are no randomized, case–control studies comparing radical vaginal trachelectomy with standard radical abdominal hysterectomy, this fertility sparing surgery is an option for patients with stage IA2 to IB1 disease. In addition, laparoscopic pelvic and para-aortic lymphadenectomy is an option for patients who are found to have unsuspected cervical cancer after a hysterectomy is performed for benign indications [31].

Several surgeons, especially in Europe, have investigated the sensitivity and specificity of sentinel lymph node mapping in cervical cancer. Plante and colleagues [33] published results in 2003 illustrating the improved sensitivity of blue dye injection in combination with radioactive technetium. A large study group (N = 70) began with only blue dye, and then converted to combined blue dye and a radioactive label when a gamma hand probe was developed for the laparoscope. With both injections, the sensitivity was 93%, positive predictive value 100%, and the a false negative rate was zero. Other authors found similar results [34,35]. Also of importance is the pathologic examination of the sentinel lymph node(s) removed, which is dependent on the pathologist. Fanfani [36] found that the accuracy of frozen section interpretations is quite high, with only 10 false negative nodes and 5 false positive lymph nodes in 2718 out of 6710 nodes submitted at one institution. This experimental procedure may one day be used to intra-operatively triage patients with positive lymph nodes to less radical surgery.

The treatment of recurrent or persistent cervical cancer is usually determined by the mode of primary therapy (surgery or radiation) and the site of recurrence. In general, patients who were initially treated with surgery should undergo radiation therapy and visa versa. For patients who are not candidates for surgical or radiation therapy, timing of second-line or palliative therapy should be individualized. In general, such patients should be encouraged to consider participation in appropriate clinical trials.

Surgery for recurrent or persistent cervical cancer is limited to patients with central pelvic disease, and is usually reserved for radiation failures. Often tumor extension to the pelvic sidewall is difficult to assess due to radiation fibrosis. In such cases, a preoperative positron emission tomogram (PET) or CT scan of the chest, abdomen, and pelvis should be obtained, and any suspicious lesions should have a needle biopsy when possible to exclude distant metastases. Some investigators advocate the use of routine scalene lymph node biopsy for all exenteration candidates because exenterative surgery is often morbid [37,38], but in the absence of suspicious nodal disease (from diagnostic image), this practice must be questioned. The efficacy of exenterative surgery for recurrent or persistent cervical cancer depends largely on judicious selection of patients: 5-year survival rates range from 6% to 74% [39].

The site of local recurrence usually dictates the surgical approach. Patients with recurrences limited to the anterior aspect of the upper vagina are suitable candidates for anterior exenteration. Posterior exenteration is indicated for patients with posterior vaginal recurrences where ureteric dissection through the cardinal ligaments is not required. Lesions involving both the anterior and posterior vagina, or those that extend into the lower vagina, may require total pelvic exenteration, with or without a perineal phase. In highly selected patients with small volume disease limited to the cervix, extrafascial or radical hysterectomy may be effective [40]. This approach has been associated with serious urinary complications when used in this setting [40,41].

Ovarian cancer

Ovarian cancer is the leading cause of death among patients with gynecologic malignancies in the United States [42]. Epithelial ovarian carcinoma is the most common ovarian malignancy and, because they usually are asymptomatic until metastases occur, approximately 60% of patients present with stage III or IV disease [1]. Initial management often encompasses complex operative procedures that require extensive knowledge of pelvic anatomy and wide-ranging surgical techniques. Because the survival is significantly longer when minimal residual disease remains after initial cytoreductive surgery, aggressive operative intervention has become accepted therapy in the early management of this disease.

Ovarian cancer is surgically staged (Table 2) based on the pattern by which it spreads. This tumor spreads primarily by direct extension and by exfoliation, and travels through ascetic fluid within the peritoneal cavity. Metastasis also occurs through the para-aortic lymph channels, and the iliac

Table 2
Ovarian cancer FIGO staging

I	Tumor limited to ovaries (one or both)
IA	Tumor limited to one ovary; capsule intact, no tumor on ovarian surface. No Malignant cells in ascites or peritoneal washings.
IB	Tumor limited to both ovaries; capsules intact, no tumor on ovarian surface. No Malignant cells in ascites or peritoneal washings.
IC	Tumor limited to one or both ovaries with any of the following: capsule ruptured, tumor on ovarian surface, malignant cells in ascites or peritoneal washings
II	Tumor involves one or both ovaries with pelvic extension and/or implants
IIA	Extension and/or implants on uterus and/or tubes (s). No malignant cells in ascites or peritoneal washings.
IIB	Extension to and/or implants on other pelvic tissues. No malignant cells in ascites or peritoneal washings.
IIC	Pelvic extension and/or implants with malignant cells in ascites or peritoneal washings.
III	Tumor involves one or both ovaries with microscopically confirmed peritoneal metastasis outside the pelvis.
IIIA	Microscopic peritoneal metastasis beyond pelvis (no macroscopic tumor)
IIIB	Macroscopic peritoneal metastasis beyond pelvis 2 cm or less in greatest dimension
IIIC	Peritoneal metastasis beyond pelvis more than 2 cm in greatest dimension and/or regional lymph node metastasis
IV	Distant metastasis (excludes peritoneal metastasis)

and inguinal lymph nodes. Surgical staging is done as follows: peritoneal washings, inspection of the tumor for rupture or excresences or adhesions, inspection of the diaphragm and Papanicolaou scraping, partial (infracolic) omentectomy, evaluation of the small and large bowel, biopsies of pelvic peritoneum, biopsy of cul-de-sac peritoneum, paraaortic lymph node sampling, and biopsies of anything suspicious [43].

Starting in 1978, Piver found that microscopic metastatsis can be found at surgery for stage I and stage II disease [44]. Before complete staging, patients with presumed stage I disease had only a 60% to 70% 5-year survival when only a total abdominal hysterectomy and bilateral salpingo-oophorectomy (TAH/BSO) was performed. The 5-year survival for presumed stage II treated with simple TAH/BSO was 40% to 50% [43]. In a landmark article from 1983, the Ovarian Cancer Study Group published the first prospective study of comprehensive surgical staging [45]. This was a multicenter consortium consisting of The Mayo Clinic, the M.D. Anderson Cancer Center, the Roswell Park Cancer Center, and the National Cancer Institute. Out of 100 patients, 31% were upstaged at surgery, and of these, 77% were upstaged to stage III.

Given the known pathway of metastasis, it was important to determine which patients with ovarian cancer would benefit from adjuvant chemotherapy. In 1990, the Ovarian Cancer Study Group published its results of 81 patients with stage Ia and Ib disease with well-differentiated or moderately well-differentiated histologic grades, who were randomized to no adjuvant therapy or melphalan. The 5-year survival rate was >90% for both groups. No benefit in disease-free survival or overall survival was seen in the melphalan group. A second study enrolled 141 patients with stage I poorly differentiated tumor or stage II disease to receive melphalan or intraperitoneal ^{32}P at the time of surgery. The 5-year survival was 80%, and about equal between the groups. Before this, 5-year survival rates for stage Ic to IIc was 40% to 60% [46]. Another study evaluated the use of cisplatin in patients with stage IC or stage I, grade 3 ovarian cancer, where 20 out of 32 patients were surgically staged. The median follow-up was 5 years, and there were three (9%) recurrences, and a 5-year progression free survival of 90.5% and overall 5-year survival of 93.3% [47]. Adjuvant chemotherapy is recommended for all ovarian cancer patients except stage IA or IB with well- or moderately well-differentated tumors.

Radical cytoreduction

Starting in 1969, Delclos and Quinlan discovered that patients in whom cytoreduction for stage III ovarian cancer achieved nonpalpable disease had a 25% 5-year survival rate versus 9% for patients in whom the cancer remained palpable [48]. In 1975, Griffiths described patients' survival with stage II or III disease as it related to residual tumor size at the end of surgery: if no gross tumor was left behind, there was a median survival of 39 months; for residual tumor >1.5 cm, the median survival was 12.7 months [49]. In other words, unless tumor was removed down to <1.5 cm, survival was not improved by surgical excision. This began the foundation for optimal debulking in ovarian cancer. In 1978, Griffiths and Fuller [50] reported that cytoreduction of the tumor to 1.0 ± 0.5 cm was associated with longer patient survival (Fig. 3). More recent studies support the role of surgical debulking in the treatment of this disease. Baker and colleagues [51], in a study of 136 patients with stage III or IV ovarian cancer treated with cytoreductive surgery followed by chemotherapy with cisplatin, doxorubicin, and cyclophosphamide, found that patients with <1 cm of residual disease after primary surgery had an improved survival compared with patients with 1 to 2 cm or greater residual disease ($P < .001$). Hoskins and colleagues [52] also found that stage III patients who had less residual disease experienced a longer survival.This study found that patients cytoreduced to <2 cm survived longer than patients with residual disease >2 cm, and that there was little survival difference between 2 and 10 cm residual disease. Currently, it is unclear whether volume of disease or overall maximal residual tumor diameter is more important in surgical debulking.

Chemotherapy

In a 1978 trial of multiagent nonplatinum chemotherapy versus single-agent alkylating chemotherapy, Young [53] observed that patients who had undergone optimal debulking had a better clinical response. This was later

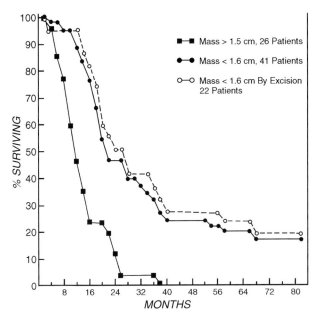

Fig. 3. Improved survival in patients cytoreduced to <1.5 cm residual disease. No difference in survival in between patients with residual disease <1.5 cm or less. (*From* Griffiths CT, Fuller AF. Intensive surgical and chemotherapeutic management of advanced ovarian cancer. Surg Clin North Am 1978;58:131–42; with permission.)

supported by Wharton and Herson [54] in 1981, and Hacker and colleaguse [55] in 1983, who also found that cytoreduction influences the success of future chemotherapy response. Omura [56], in 1987, using a Gynecologic Oncology Group (GOG) protocol comparing two cisplatin-based regimens, found once again that patients who had no gross residual disease had a statistically significant progression-free interval and overall survival advantage. Last, in 1994, Baker, Piver, and Hempling [51] found that optimal debulking improved patient response to chemotherapy and overall survival.

Current therapy for ovarian cancer is based on these studies. The goals of surgery are to accurately stage patients and to optimize cytoreduction of the tumor burden.

Patients with stage I disease should undergo complete surgical staging with a TAH/BSO, infracolic omentectomy, diaphragmatic scraping, peritoneal biopsies, and pelvic and para-aortic lymphadenectomy. In addition, peritoneal washings should be taken at the beginning of surgery. Attention is focused particularly on the sites where ovarian malignancies typically spread: the leaves of the diaphragms, the capsule of the liver, the omentum, the parietal peritoneum, the mesentery of the large and small intestine, and the retroperitoneal lymph nodes. An infracolic omentectomy is performed by ligating and dividing the branches of the gastroepiploic vessels along the transverse colon. Pelvic and para-aortic lymph nodes should be inspected, and enlarged nodal tissue should be resected. In the absence of gross evidence of upper abdominal disease, para-aortic nodal sampling is indicated. Finally, the pelvic structures are scrutinized, and the primary tumor should be resected and sent for frozen section to facilitate the subsequent surgical management of the remaining pelvic organs and to aid in assessing the value of additional tumor debulking efforts.

Although fertility sparing surgery with simple unilateral salpino-oophorectomy can be performed for stage I disease, the recurrence rate is 20% [57]. Stage II disease requires TAH/BSO, omentectomy, and lympha-denectomy. Stage III disease staging is determined by extent of disease. For stage IIIa and stage IIIb disease (ie, microscopic metastasis or omental lesions <2 cm) a lymphadenectomy is performed. For stage IIIc or stage IV disease surgical efforts are aimed at reducing tumor load by performing a maximal debulking effort to remove all tumor to less than 1 cm.

The upper extent of surgical resection for ovarian cancer includes large and small bowel resection, liver resection, splenectomy, and diaphragmatic resection.

Cytoreductive surgery

An extended midline abdominal incision assures adequate exposure for cytoreductive procedures. Patients with advanced stage disease often have an "omental cake," where tumor involves the entire omentum. In such cases, a total, supracolic, omentectomy is indicated. Beginning at the hepatic flexure of the large intestine, the omentum is dissected free from the transverse colon by clamping and ligating vascular branches of the right gastroepiploic artery. The omentum is separated from the greater curvature of the stomach by ligating vascular contributions from the short gastric and the right and left gastroepiploic vessels. Automated surgical staplers, such as the linear dis-section stapler (LDS), can expedite this portion of the operation.

Resection of the primary ovarian tumor frequently presents a challenge because the mass is often sizable, there can be extensive adhesive disease, and there is distortion of normal anatomy. It is helpful to dissect the peritoneum laterally, allowing entry into the retroperitoneum where anatomic landmarks can be identified more readily. Division and ligation of the round ligament bilaterally aids in the retroperitoneal dissection by furnishing a relatively fibrous structure to use for countertraction. The anterior and posterior leaves of the broad ligament are incised, and the iliac vessels and ureter are identified after careful blunt dissection. The pararectal and paravesical spaces are opened. Next, the infundibulopelvic ligament, which contains the ovarian vessels, is visualized, skeletonized, then double clamped, double ligated, and divided. A bladder flap is developed by connecting the anterior incisions of the broad ligament bilaterally, then the bladder is mobilized free from the anterior cervix and vagina using careful sharp dissection.

Hysterectomy is performed by skeletonizing the uterine vessels, clamping, and ligating them. Then, in a stepwise fashion and alternating from side to side, the parametrial and paracervical tissues are clamped, cut, and ligated to the vaginal angles, which are crossclamped, cut, and ligated. The bladder is advanced accordingly, and the ureters are kept in view throughout this part of the operation. The cervix is transected free from the vagina, allowing removal of the tumor, the uterus, and the cervix; then the mucosa of the vaginal cuff is approximated with suture ligatures.

Occasionally, the tumor may obscure the ureters when approached cephalically. In such instances, a retrograde approach is employed wherein the bladder is mobilized free of the cervix, and the ureters are unroofed from the overlying cardinal ligaments and dissected cephalad until the uterine vessels are encountered near their origin at the hypogastric artery and vein. Additionally, malignancy may encase the cul-de-sac of Douglas and preclude isolation of the cervix from the underlying rectum. A suitable option is to perform a supracervical hysterectomy by transecting the uterine fundus at the level of the cervical isthmus after the uterine vessels have been ligated. En block resection of the rectosigmoid colon along with the uterus and cervix is another alternative when the aim is to achieve minimal residual disease at the conclusion of the operation. This is accomplished by developing the pararectal space, mobilizing the colonic mesentery just proximal to the extent of disease involvement, then clamping across the mesentery to permit division of the colon and removal of the involved bowel. Transection of the lower uterine segment or vagina may permit access to an uninvolved portion of the rectum, which may be divided with stapling devices, thereby allowing the rectosigmoid to be removed in continuity with the cul-de-sac peritoneum, uterus, ovaries, and fallopian tubes. Frequently, primary low rectal anastomoses can be achieved with the aid of the end-to-end anastomosis (EEA) stapling device, although it may be necessary at times to create an end colostomy when there is insufficient residual rectal length. On rare occasion, a part of the bladder may require resection. In such instances, an intentional cystotomy will frequently afford advantageous exposure and permit effective resection and surgical repair. Management of ureteral injury or resection largely depends on the location of the segment involved and the length of the remaining ureter. Surgical options include primary ureteral reanastomosis, ureteroneocystotomy, or transureteroureterostomy.

Endometrial cancer

Endometrial cancer is the most common malignancy of the female reproductive tract, with an estimated 40,000 new cases and 7000 deaths in the United States in 2004 [42]. The peak incidence of endometrial cancer is at age 63, and malignancies in patients less than 40 years of age are relatively uncommon. Ninety-seven percent of all cancers of the uterine corpus arise from the glands of the endometrium; uterine sarcomas account for the remaining 3%. Uterine sarcomas are detected and treated in a manner similar to endometrial cancers, but the intensity of initial surgery and the recommended chemotherapeutic agents may differ depending upon the histologic type of tumor, the stage, the grade, and the depth of myometrial invasion.

Endometrial cancer, like ovarian cancer, is staged surgically. In 1988, FIGO developed the current staging of endometrial cancer, replacing the clinical staging system developed in 1976 (Table 3). In the 1980s, Cowles and colleagues [58] stated that the clinical staging of endometrial cancer was grossly inaccurate. In his study of 62 patients, 52% had the stage changed after surgery, and 33.8% of the patients had the tumor grade changed. Today, the surgical approach is based on the metastatic pathway of the tumor that spreads to the paracervical and parametrial lymphatics, ovarian lymphatics, and round ligament lymphatics.

Also of importance is the direct spread of tumor from its primary source in the endometrium through the myometrium. Currently, the most important prognostic factors for endometrial cancer are size and volume of tumor, cervical involvement, depth of myometrial invasion; cell type, DNA ploidy, histologic grading; nodal status, extrauterine spread; lymphovascular invasion; positive peritoneal washings, and the estrogen/progesterone status of the tumor.

History

Like cervical cancer, endometrial cancer was treated with radiation therapy during the first half of the twentieth century. In current practice,

Table 3
Endometrial cancer FIGO staging

0	Carcinoma in situ
I	Tumor confined to corpus uteri
IA	Tumor limited to endometrium
IB	Tumor invades less than one-half of the myometrium
IC	Tumor invades one-half or more of the myometrium
II	Tumor invades cervix but does not extend beyond uterus
IIA	Tumor limited to the glandular epithelium of the endocervix. There is no evidence of connective tissue stromal invasion.
IIB	Invasion of the stromal connective tissue of the cervix.
III	Local and/or regional spread as defined below
IIIA	Tumor involves serosa and/or adnexa (direct extension or metastasis) and/or cancer cells in ascitses or peritoneal washings
IIIB	Vaginal involvement (direct extension or metastasis)
IIIC	Regional lymph node metastasis to pelvic and/or para-aortic nodes
IVA	Tumor invades bladder mucosa and/or bowel mucosa
IVB	Distant metastasis (includes metastasis to abdominal lymph nodes other than para-aortic, and/or inguinal lymph nodes; excludes metastasis to vagina, pelvic serosa, or adnexa)

primary radiation therapy is reserved for women who are considered medically inoperable because of serious medical problems, morbid obesity, or very elderly patients. Such patients account for less than 10% of patients with endometrial cancer [59]. When treatment for clinical stage I disease included both external beam irradiation and intracavitary radiotherapy, survival rates of 94% for grade 1, 92% for grade 2, and 78% for grade 3 tumors have been reported [60].

Currently, stage I disease is treated with a TAH/BSO. The incidence of lymph node metastases correlates with the grade of the tumor and its depth of myometrial invasion [61]; therefore, pelvic and para-aortic lymph node sampling is suggested for all grade 3 lesions, also for any tumors with invasion into the middle third of the myometrium, when tumor extends into the endocervix, and for papillary-serous or clear cell histologies [62]. Papillary serous lesions have a propensity for extrauterine metastases with relatively poor overall survival [63,64].

Clear cell carcinoma, a more aggressive cell type, usually occurs in older women [65]. Intraoperatively, the uterus should be opened following its removal and inspected by a pathologist to assess the degree of myometrial invasion. For grade 1 tumors, gross examination can accurately predict the depth of myometrial invasion in almost 90% of cases [66]. Patients with grade 1 or 2 lesions with only superficial myometrial invasion are at low risk of nodal metastases and may be spared the risks nodal sampling [61].

There is continued debate about whether to perform a complete lymphadenectomy or a lymph node sampling at the time of surgical staging. Authors have found that lymphadenectomy both identifies low-risk patients with lymph node metastases and avoids postoperative radiation of high-risk patients in whom there are no lymph node metastases [67,68]. GOG protocol 33 found that patients with stage I or II were more likely to have lymph node metastases with higher grade tumor and increasing depth of invasion. The results of this study suggested that patients with grade 1 tumors limited to the endometrium need not undergo lymphadenectomy [61]. However, tumor grade may be changed with the surgical specimen. Goudge and colleagues [69] published a study in 2004 supporting complete surgical staging with pelvic and para-aortic lymphadenectomy for patients with endometrial cancer. They found that 50 tumors out of 285 patients (18%) had a final surgical grade greater than the preoperative grade, 45 (17%) patients had positive nodes, and of these patients 23 had both pelvic and para-aortic nodal metastases. Patients who are treated with a complete lymphadenectomy at the time of surgery do very well without postoperative radiation. Straughn and colleagues [70], in 2002, published a retrospective review of 613 patients who underwent comprehensive surgical staging with pelvic/para-aortic lymphadenectomy. There were 325 stage IB patients, 321 of whom did not receive adjuvant radiation. Of the 5% in whom cancer recurred, nine were local and the patients were salvaged with whole pelvic radiation and brachytherapy. Of the 77 patients with stage IC, 69% had no adjuvant therapy, and 8% recurred. Overall, the 5-year disease free survival was 93%, and the overall 5-year survival was 98%, supporting surgical staging followed by conservative management.

Also supporting lymphadenectomy is the finding that no survival advantage has been shown in patients who receive postoperative radiation. In a prospective, multicenter randomized trial of patients treated only with TAH/BSO, it was found that postoperative radiotherapy reduced local recurrence, but had no impact on overall survival for stage I disease [71]. In addition, patients who received radiation had a higher rate of complications due to treatment (25% versus 6%, $P < .0001$) [71]. Currently, lympha-denectomy should be performed when there is greater than 50% myometrial invasion; extension to cervical isthmus; adnexa/extrauterine extension; cell type of clear serous, undifferentiated, or squamous. Gynecologic oncologists have argued that complete surgical staging should be performed in all endometrial cancer cases [72]. Surgical staging may be done by either a lymph node sampling or complete lymphadenectomy for stage I endometrial cancer, and postoperative radiation may be called for by the pathologic findings of the surgical specimen.

Stage II disease is suspected before surgery if there is evidence of cervical invasion, either detected during pelvic examination or with fractional D&C, or by an imaging modality such as ultrasound, MRI, or hysteroscopy. Treatment consists of a TAH/BSO/pelvic and para-aortic lymphadenectomy with the submission of a peritoneal washing sample. The role for radical hysterectomy is unclear in stage II disease, as there is no data supporting direct spread to the parametria in endometrial cancer. Occasionally, a radical or modified radical hysterectomy is necessary to resect large primary endometrial lesions involving the lower uterine segment.

Stage III and stage IV endometrial cancer, due to its extensive anatomical involvement, is considered by many to be surgically incurable; however, it is often palliated with radiation therapy, and some surgeons have supported surgical management [73].

In cases where cancer is unexpectedly found after a hysterectomy, laparoscopic lymphadenectomy can be performed for endometrial cancer, thus allowing a patient to undergo complete staging without a laparotomy [74].

Vulvar cancer

Vulvar cancer accounts for 3% to 5% of all gynecologic cancer cases. In 2004, there were an estimated 3970 new cases in the United States and 850 deaths [42]. This disease is staged surgically, and the FIGO staging system was changed in 1995 to include surgical assessment of groin nodes (Table 4). The lymphatic drainage of the vulva is primarily ipsilateral, with the dermal lymphatics traveling to the mons pubis and then draining into the superficial lymph nodes [75]. From there, the lymphatics drain into the deep inguinal

Table 4
Vulvar cancer FIGO staging

0	Carcinoma in situ (preinvasive carcinoma)
I	Tumor confined to the vulva or vulva and perineum, 2 cm or less in greatest dimension
IA	Tumor confined to the vulva or vulva and perineum, 2 cm or less in greatest dimension, and with stromal invasion no greater than 1 mm
IB	Tumor confined to the vulva or vulva and perineum 2 cm or less in greatest dimension, and with stromal invasion greater than 1 mm
II	Tumor confined to the vulva or vulva and perineum, more than 2 cm in greatest dimension
III	Tumor of any size with contiguous spread to the lower urethra and/or vagina or anus or unilateral regional lymph node metastasis
IVA	Tumor invades any of the following: upper urethra, bladder mucosa, rectal mucosa, or is fixed to the pubic bone or bilateral regional lymh node metastasis
IVB	Distant metastasis (including pelvic lymph node metastasis)

nodes below the cribiform fascia. At the midline of the vulva there is bilateral lymphatic drainage, as suggested by Stanley Way [76] (Fig. 4). This understanding of the lymphatic drainage of the vulva has directed surgical treatment of vulvar cancer.

Historically, vulvar cancer has been treated with radical surgery that was often quite disfiguring. In the 1950s and 1960s, en bloc radical vulvectomy was developed. The vulva was removed in conjunction with a bilateral inguinofemoral lymphadenectomy, via either a "butterfly" or "longhorn" approach (Fig. 5). This resulted in long term survival and local control in close to 90% of patients [77], but the rate of wound disruption was 40% [78]. The cosmetic outcome was poor, and the effects on a woman's sexual function were devastating. This fueled a movement toward less mutilating

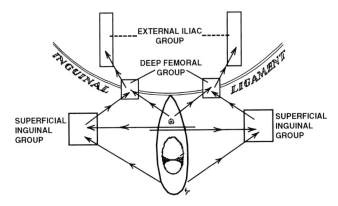

Fig. 4. Stanley Way's representation of the lymphatic spread of vulvar cancer. (*From* Way S. Malignant disease of the female genital tract. London: Churchill Livingstone; 1951, as cited in Hoskins WJ, Perez CA, Young RC, editors. Principles and practice of gynecologic oncology. 4th edition. Philadelphia: Lippincott-Raven; 2005. p. 672; with permission.)

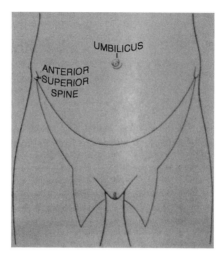

Fig. 5. Butterfly incision with en bloc resection of vulva and inguinal lymphatics. (*From* Way S. Malignant disease of the female genital tract. London: Churchill Livingstone, 1951; with permission.)

radical surgery, beginning in the 1960s with Byron and colleagues [79–82] proposing a radical vulvectomy with groin dissection completed through three incisions in the perineum. DiSaia and colleagues [83] first described conservative resection of tumors 1 cm or less with a depth of invasion of less than 5 mm. Eighteen patients underwent a wide local excision and bilateral superficial inguinal lymphadenectomy, and in mean follow-up of 32 months (range 7–74) there were no recurrences (see Fig. 6 for vulvectomy modifications).

Over time, the risk factors associated with groin metastases were understood. In 1971, Franklin and Rutledge [84] thought that patients with ≤5 mm invasion had no risk of groin involvement. However, later studies found that patients with stage I disease with stromal invasion of 5 mm or less did indeed have groin node metastases. In a review of 77 patients with stage I disease with a depth of invasion of 5 mm or less, the following results were found: depth of invasion of 1 mm or less, none of 34 patients had positive lymph nodes; 1.1 to 2 mm, 2 of 19 had positive lymph nodes; 2.1 to 3 mm, two of 17 had positive lymph nodes; 3 to 5 mm, one of seven had positive lymph nodes; >5 mm, three of seven had positive lymph nodes [85]. A prospective GOG study investigated factors that would predict groin node metastases in squamous cell carcinoma. Of 588 patients included in the study, 477 had palpably normal inguinal lymph nodes. However, surgical specimens showed metastases in 23.9% of these patients, once again supporting that clinical assessment of the groin is inadequate. The study also found that the risk of groin metastases increased with increasing tumor depth, and that 20.6% of patients with lesions ≤5 mm had positive groin

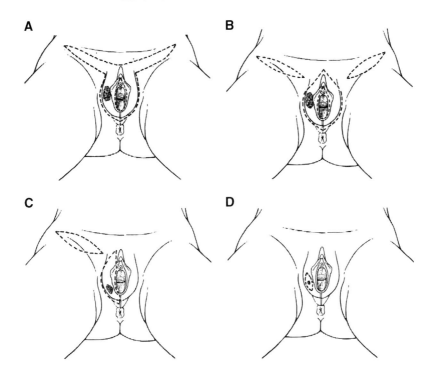

Fig. 6. Modifications of vulvectomy/lymphadenectomy (*A*,*B*,*C*,*D*). (*From* Rock JA, Thomspon JD, editors. TeLinde's operative gynecology. 8th edition. Philadelphia: Lippincott, Williams & Wilkins; 1997; with permission.)

nodes. Increasing tumor size correlated with increased risk of groin metastases, with tumors <1 cm and tumors 1.1 to 2 cm each having <20% occurrence of groin nodes, whereas tumors 2.1 to >5 cm having 31.4% to 51.8% occurrence of positive groin [86].

Current treatment of vulvar cancer is based on the size of the tumor, depth of invasion, location of the tumor relative to the midline, and suspicious groin nodes. The goal of removing as much tumor as possible, while producing a more cosmetic result, has driven individualized surgical procedures. For a stage IA vulvar cancer, a wide local excision is curative. Studies have found that an inguinofemoral lymphadenectomy can be omitted when the tumor depth of invasion is ≤1 mm. Any greater depth of invasion carries an increased risk of lymph node metastases. For tumors >1 cm from the midline, radical wide local excision of the primary tumor and only an ipsilateral lymphadenectomy is necessary. The lymphadenectomy should include at least all the medial femoral lymph nodes and all the superficial lymph nodes. Because of the possibility of bilateral lymphatic drainage, tumors <1 cm from the midline require bilateral inguinal lymphadenectomy. However, there is concern that lymphatic drainage is altered in the presence of nodal metastases [87]. Because of this, some surgeons argue that when more than one lymph node is positive for metastases, the contralateral groin should be treated with either lymphadenectomy or radiation.

Another concern with the three incision technique is the possibility of recurrence in the skin between the incisions, also known as skin bridge recurrence [82,88,89]. In 1989, Hacker reviewed the literature and found that local recurrence after radical local excision was comparable to radical vulvectomy (5.3% versus 8.1%) [90]. In 2002, de Hullu and colleagues [91] reported outcomes for treatment with radical vulvectomy with en bloc inguinofemoral lymphadenectomy or with wide local excision and lymphadenectomy through separate incisions. A total of 253 patients were treated, and although survival was comparable, recurrence in the wide local excision cohort was significantly higher (33.3% versus 19.9%, $P = .03$), as was the development of fatal groin or skin bridge recurrence (6.3% versus 1.3%, $P = .029$) De Hullu has recommended that only patients who have suspicious inguinofemoral lymph nodes should undergo an en bloc excision to decrease the possibility of skin bridge recurrences [92].

For stages II and III, a radical vulvectomy is performed, where the goal is to have a 2-cm surgical margin around the tumor. If necessary, the distal 2 cm of the urethra can be resected without compromising continence. For stage IV tumors, a pelvic exenteration can be performed, and if necessary, a colostomy. Recently, neoadjuvant chemotherapy using cisplatin and 5-fluorouracil has been used in nine patients with locally advanced vulvar carcinoma involving the urethra or anal sphincter [93]. All nine patients (100%) responded positively to neoadjuvant chemotherapy and subsequently underwent radical vulvectomy in which the anal or urethral sphincter was preserved. In two patients, there was no residual invasive carcinoma on final pathology.

Over the last 10 years, surgeons have investigated the use of sentinel node mapping in vulvar cancer. Levenback published the first study using isosulfan blue in a small series of patients in 1994 [94]. Since then it has been discovered that combining the blue dye intraoperatively with a radioactive tracer with preoperative lymphoscintoigraphy results in a high identification rate [92]. Currently, a prospective Gynecologic Oncology Group trial (GOG study 173) is addressing the use of the sentinel lymph node procedure in patients with vulvar cancer.

Summary

Surgical treatment of gynecologic malignancies has developed rapidly over the last century. Surgical management has been adapted to growth in understanding of tumor behavior. Radical surgery still is the basis for diagnosis and therapy in endometrial, ovarian, and vulvar cancer. Clinical staging still is used in cervical cancer, but radical surgery plays a key role in therapy. As surgeons come to understand the risks and benefits of surgical, chemotherapeutic, and radiation therapeutic modalities, the multimodal approach to gynecologic cancer will evolve. Future research in sentinel lymph node mapping may allow patients to undergo less morbid procedures, and may limit unwanted side effects in cervical and vulvar cancers. As data on radical trachelectomy continues to accrue, more young women diagnosed with cervical cancer may retain their reproductive capacities. Although cytoreductive surgery has been an important step in ovarian cancer, future work in immunology and pharmacology may improve treatment of this often fatal disease.

References

[1] Pisani P, Parkin DM, Bray F, et al. Estimates of the worldwide mortality from 25 cancers in 1990. Int J Cancer 1999;83(1):18–29.

[2] Piver MS. Handbook of gynecologic oncology. Boston: Little, Brown and Company; 1996.

[3] Kurman RJ, Henson DE, Herbst AL, et al. Interim guidelines for management of abnormal cervical cytology. The 1992 National Cancer Institute Workshop. JAMA 1994;271:1866–9.

[4] Cates W Jr. Estimates of the incidence and prevalence of sexually transmitted diseases in the United States. American Social Health Association Panel. Sex Transm Dis 1999;26(4 Suppl): S2–7.

[5] Walboomers JM, Jacobs MV, Manos MM, et al. Human papillomavirus is a necessary cause of invasive cervical cancer worldwide. J Pathol 1999;189(1):12–9.

[6] Shingleton HM, Thompson JD. Cancer of the cervix. In: Rock JA, Thompson JD, editors. TeLinde's operative gynecology. Philadelphia: Lippincott Williams & Wilkins; 1997. p. 1413–500.

[7] Zweifel P. Zum Ancleken an die erste Totalexstirpation des Karzinomaatosen uterus. Much Med Wochem 1922;69:19.

[8] Freund W. Zu meiner Methode der totalen Uterus-Exstirpation. Z Gynakol 1878;2:265.

[9] Linkenheld J. Zur Totalexstirpation des Uterus. Z Gynakol 1881;5:169.

[10] Clark J. A more radical method of performing hysterectomy for cancer of the uterus. Bull Johns Hopkins Hosp 1895;6:120.

[11] Meigs J. Carcinoma of the cervix: the Wertheim operation. Surg Gynecol Obstet 1944;78: 195.

[12] Cruveilhier J. Traite d'anatomie descriptive. Paris: Bechet Jeune; 1834.

[13] Wagner N. Eine pathologisch-anatomische Monographie. Leipzig; 1858.

[14] Latzko W, Schiffmann J. Klinisches und Anatomisches zur Radikaloperation des Gebarmutterkrebses. Zbl Gynakol 1919;34:689–705.

[15] Peiser E. Anatomische und lkinische Untersuchungen uber den Lymphapparat des Uterus mit besonderer Berucksichtigung der Totalexstirpation bei Carcinoma uteri. Z Geburtshilfe Gynakol 1898;39:259–78.

[16] Bonney V. The results of 500 cases of Wertheim's operation for carcinoma of the cervix. J Obstet Gynaecol Br Emp 1941;48:421.

[17] Piver MS, Rutledge F, Smith JP. Five classes of extended hysterectomy for women with cervical cancer. Obstet Gynecol 1974;44(2):265–72.

[18] Stehman F, Perez C, Kurman R, et al. Uterine cervix. In: Hoskins W, Perez C, Young R, editors. Principles and practice of gynecologic oncology. Philadelphia: Lippincot-Raven; 1997. p. 785–858.

[19] Cervical Cancer. NIH consensus statement 1996. Bethesda (MD): NIH; 14(1):1–38.

[20] Benedet JL, Anderson GH. Stage IA carcinoma of the cervix revisited. Obstet Gynecol 1996; 87(6):1052–9.

[21] US Dept of Health and Human Services. NCI clinical announcement. Bethesda (MD): Public Health Service, National Institutes of Health; 1999.

[22] Whitney CW, Sause W, Bundy BN, et al. Randomized comparison of fluorouracil plus cisplatin versus hydroxyurea as an adjunct to radiation therapy in stage IIB–IVA carcinoma of the cervix with negative para-aortic lymph nodes: a Gynecologic Oncology Group and Southwest Oncology Group study. J Clin Oncol 1999;17(5):1339–48.

[23] Morris M, Eifel PJ, Lu J, et al. Pelvic radiation with concurrent chemotherapy compared with pelvic and para-aortic radiation for high-risk cervical cancer. N Engl J Med 1999; 340(15):1137–43.

[24] Rose PG, Bundy BN, Watkins EB, et al. Concurrent cisplatin-based radiotherapy and chemotherapy for locally advanced cervical cancer. N Engl J Med 1999;340(15):1144–53.

[25] Peters WA III, Liu PY, Barrett RJ, et al. Concurrent chemotherapy and pelvic radiation therapy compared with pelvic radiation therapy alone as adjuvant therapy after radical surgery in high-risk early-stage cancer of the cervix. J Clin Oncol 2000;18(8):1606–13.

[26] Keys HM, Bundy BN, Stehman FB, et al. Cisplatin, radiation, and adjuvant hysterectomy compared with radiation and adjuvant hysterectomy for bulky stage IB cervical carcinoma. N Engl J Med 1999;340(15):1154–61.

[27] Green J, Kirwan J, Tierney J, et al. Concomitant chemotherapy and radiation therapy for cancer of the uterine cervix. The Cochrance Database of Systematic Reviews 3. 11–18–2003. The Cochrane Collaboration.

[28] Dargent D, Martin X, Sacchetoni A, et al. Laparoscopic vaginal radical trachelectomy: a treatment to preserve the fertility of cervical carcinoma patients. Cancer 2000;88(8): 1877–82.

[29] Koliopoulos G, Sotiriadis A, Kyrgiou M, et al. Conservative surgical methods for FIGO stage IA2 squamous cervical carcinoma and their role in preserving women's fertility. Gynecol Oncol 2004;93(2):469–73.

[30] Querleu D. Laparoscopically assisted radical vaginal hysterectomy. Gynecol Oncol 1993; 51(2):248–54.

[31] Querleu D. Laparoscopic paraaortic node sampling in gynecologic oncology: a preliminary experience. Gynecol Oncol 1993;49(1):24–9.

[32] Childers JM. Operative laparoscopy in gynaecological oncology. Baillieres Clin Obstet Gynaecol 1994;8(4):831–49.

[33] Plante M, Renaud MC, Tetu B, et al. Laparoscopic sentinel node mapping in early-stage cervical cancer. Gynecol Oncol 2003;91(3):494–503.

[34] Buist MR, Pijpers RJ, van Lingen A, et al. Laparoscopic detection of sentinel lymph nodes followed by lymph node dissection in patients with early stage cervical cancer. Gynecol Oncol 2003;90(2):290–6.

[35] Martinez-Palones JM, Gil-Moreno A, Perez-Benavente MA, et al. Intraoperative sentinel node identification in early stage cervical cancer using a combination of radiolabeled albumin injection and isosulfan blue dye injection. Gynecol Oncol 2004;92(3):845–50.

[36] Fanfani F, Ludovisi M, Zannoni GF, et al. Frozen section examination of pelvic lymph nodes in endometrial and cervical cancer: accuracy in patients submitted to neoadjuvant treatments. Gynecol Oncol 2004;94(3):779–84.

[37] Ketcham AS, Chretien PB, Hoye RC, et al. Occult metastases to the scalene lymph nodes in patients with clinically operable carcinoma of the cervix. Cancer 1973;31: 180–3.

[38] Buchsbaum HJ, Lifshitz S. The role of scalene lymph node biopsy in advanced carcinoma of the cervix uteri. Surg Gynecol Obstet 1976;143:246–8.

[39] Shingleton HM, Orr JW. Cancer of the cervix. Philadelphia: Lippincott; 1995.

[40] Rubin SC, Hoskins WJ, Lewis JL Jr. Radical hysterectomy for recurrent cervical cancer following radiation therapy. Gynecol Oncol 1987;27:316–24.

[41] Mikuta JJ, Giuntoli RL, Rubin EL, et al. The "problem" radical hysterectomy. Am J Obstet Gynecol 1977;128:119–27.

[42] Jemal A, Clegg LX, Ward E, et al. Annual report to the nation on the status of cancer, 1975–2001, with a special feature regarding survival. Cancer 2004;101(1):3–27.

[43] Young RC. Initial therapy for early ovarian carcinoma. Cancer 1987;60(8 Suppl):2042–9.

[44] Piver MS, Barlow JJ, Lele SB. Incidence of subclinical metastasis in stage I and II ovarian carcinoma. Obstet Gynecol 1978;52(1):100–4.

[45] Young RC, Decker DG, Wharton JT, et al. Staging laparotomy in early ovarian cancer. JAMA 1983;250(22):3072–6.

[46] Young RC, Walton LA, Ellenberg SS, et al. Adjuvant therapy in stage I and stage II epithelial ovarian cancer. Results of two prospective randomized trials. N Engl J Med 1990; 322(15):1021–7.

[47] Piver MS, Malfetano J, Baker TR, et al. Five-year survival for stage IC or stage I grade 3 epithelial ovarian cancer treated with cisplatin-based chemotherapy. Gynecol Oncol 1992; 46(3):357–60.

[48] Delclos L, Quilan E. Malignant tumors of the ovary managed with postoperative megavoltage irradiation. Radiology 1969;93:659.

[49] Griffiths C. Surgical resection of tumor bulk in the primary treatment of ovarian carcinoma. Natl Cancer Inst Monogr 1975;42:101–4.

[50] Griffiths C, Fuller A. Intensive surgical and chemotherapeutic management of advanced ovarian cancer. Surg Clin North Am 1978;58(1):131–42.

[51] Baker TR, Piver MS, Hempling RE. Long term survival by cytoreductive surgery to less than 1 cm, induction weekly cisplatin and monthly cisplatin, doxorubicin, and cyclophosphamide therapy in advanced ovarian adenocarcinoma. Cancer 1994;74(2):656–63.

[52] Hoskins WJ, McGuire WP, Brady MF, et al. The effect of diameter of largest residual disease on survival after primary cytoreductive surgery in patients with suboptimal residual epithelial ovarian carcinoma. Am J Obstet Gynecol 1994;170(4):974–9.

[53] Young RC, Chabner BA, Hubbard SP, et al. Advanced ovarian adenocarcinoma. A prospective clinical trial of melphalan. (L-PAM) versus combination chemotherapy. N Engl J Med 1978;299(23):1261–6.

[54] Wharton JT, Herson J. Surgery for common epithelial tumors of the ovary. Cancer 1981; 48(2 Suppl):582–9.

[55] Hacker NF, Berek JS, Lagasse LD, et al. Primary cytoreductive surgery for epithelial ovarian cancer. Obstet Gynecol 1983;61(4):413–20.

[56] Omura G, Blessing JA, Ehrlich CE, et al. A randomized trial of cyclophosphamide and doxorubicin with or without cisplatin in advanced ovarian carcinoma. A Gynecologic Oncology Group Study. Cancer 1986;57(9):1725–30.

[57] Burghardt E. Epithelial ovarian cancer. In: Burghard E, Webb M, Monaghan J, Kindermann G, editors. Surgical gynecologic oncology. New York: Georg Thieme Verlag; 1993. p. 457–64.

[58] Cowles TA, Magrina JF, Masterson BJ, et al. Comparison of clinical and surgical-staging in patients with endometrial carcinoma. Obstet Gynecol 1985;66(3):413–6.

[59] Varia M, Rosenman J, Halle J, et al. Primary radiation therapy for medically inoperable patients with endometrial carcinoma—stages I–II. Int J Radiat Oncol Biol Phys 1987;13(1): 11–5.

[60] Grigsby PW, Kuske RR, Perez CA, et al. Medically inoperable stage I adenocarcinoma of the endometrium treated with radiotherapy alone. Int J Radiat Oncol Biol Phys 1987;13(4): 483–8.

[61] Creasman WT, Morrow CP, Bundy BN, et al. Surgical pathologic spread patterns of endometrial cancer. A Gynecologic Oncology Group Study. Cancer 1987;60(8 Suppl): 2035–41.

[62] American College of Obstetricians and Gynecologists. Carcinoma of the endometrium. Washington (DC): The American College of Obstetricians and Gynecologists. ACOG

Technical Bulletin. Committee on Technical Bulletins of the American College of Obstetricians and Gynecologists; 1991. p. 1–6.

[63] Goff BA, Kato D, Schmidt RA, et al. Uterine papillary serous carcinoma: patterns of metastatic spread. Gynecol Oncol 1994;54(3):264–8.

[64] Hendrickson M, Ross J, Eifel P. Uterine papillary serous carcinoma: a highly malignant form of endometrial adenocarcinoma. Am J Surg Pathol 1982;6(2):93–108.

[65] Kurman RJ, Scully RE. Clear cell carcinoma of the endometrium: an analysis of 21 cases. Cancer 1976;37(2):872–82.

[66] Goff BA, Rice LW. Assessment of depth of myometrial invasion in endometrial adenocarcinoma. Gynecol Oncol 1990;38(1):46–8.

[67] Watanabe M, Aoki Y, Kase H, et al. Low risk endometrial cancer: a study of pelvic lymph node metastasis. Int J Gynecol Cancer 2003;13(1):38–41.

[68] Horowitz N, Powell M, Smith J, et al. Staging grade I endometrial cancers: saving dollars and lives. Proc ASCO 2003;22:1835.

[69] Goudge C, Bernhard S, Cloven NG, et al. The impact of complete surgical staging on adjuvant treatment decisions in endometrial cancer. Gynecol Oncol 2004;93(2):536–9.

[70] Straughn JM Jr, Huh WK, Kelly FJ, et al. Conservative management of stage I endometrial carcinoma after surgical staging. Gynecol Oncol 2002;84(2):194–200.

[71] Creutzberg CL, van Putten WL, Koper PC, et al. Surgery and postoperative radiotherapy versus surgery alone for patients with stage-1 endometrial carcinoma: multicentre randomised trial. PORTEC Study Group. Post Operative Radiation Therapy in Endometrial Carcinoma. Lancet 2000;355(9213):1404–11.

[72] Orr JW Jr, Roland PY, Leichter D, et al. Endometrial cancer: is surgical staging necessary? Curr Opin Oncol 2001;13(5):408–12.

[73] Goff BA, Goodman A, Muntz HG, et al. Surgical stage IV endometrial carcinoma: a study of 47 cases. Gynecol Oncol 1994;52(2):237–40.

[74] Childers JM, Spirtos NM, Brainard P, et al. Laparoscopic staging of the patient with incompletely staged early adenocarcinoma of the endometrium. Obstet Gynecol 1994;83(4): 597–600.

[75] Parry-Jones E. Lymphatics of the vulva. J Obstet Gyne Br Empire 1963;70:751.

[76] Way S. Malignant disease of the femal genital tract. London: Churchill Livingstone; 1951.

[77] Podratz KC, Symmonds RE, Taylor WF, et al. Carcinoma of the vulva: analysis of treatment and survival. Obstet Gynecol 1983;61(1):63–74.

[78] Monaghan J. Complications in the surgical management of gynaecological and obstetrical malignancy. London: Baillere Tindall; 1989.

[79] Byron R, Lamb E, Yonemotot R, et al. Radical inguinal node dissection in the treatment of cancer. Surge Gynecol Obstet 1962;114(401).

[80] Ballon SC, Lamb EJ. Separate inguinal incisions in the treatment of carcinoma of the vulva. Surg Gynecol Obstet 1975;140(1):81–4.

[81] Hoffman MS, Roberts WS, LaPolla JP, et al. Recent modifications in the treatment of invasive squamous cell carcinoma of the vulva. Obstet Gynecol Surv 1989;44(4):227–33.

[82] Grimshaw RN, Murdoch JB, Monaghan JM. Radical vulvectomy and bilateral inguinal-femoral lymphadenectomy through separate incisions-experience with 100 cases. Int J Gynecol Cancer 1993;3(1):18–23.

[83] DiSaia PJ, Creasman WT, Rich WM. An alternate approach to early cancer of the vulva. Am J Obstet Gynecol 1979;133(7):825–32.

[84] Franklin EW III, Rutledge FD. Prognostic factors in epidermoid carcinoma of the vulva. Obstet Gynecol 1971;37(6):892–901.

[85] Hacker NF, Berek JS, Lagasse LD, et al. Individualization of treatment for stage I squamous cell vulvar carcinoma. Obstet Gynecol 1984;63(2):155–62.

[86] Homesley HD, Bundy BN, Sedlis A, et al. Prognostic factors for groin node metastasis in squamous cell carcinoma of the vulva (a Gynecologic Oncology Group study). Gynecol Oncol 1993;49(3):279–83.

[87] Burger M, Hollema H, Bouma J. The side of groin node metastases in unilateral vulvar carcinoma. Int J Gynecol Cancer 1996;6:318–22.

[88] Schulz MJ, Penalver M. Recurrent vulvar carcinoma in the intervening tissue bridge in early invasive stage I disease treated by radical vulvectomy and bilateral groin dissection through separate incisions. Gynecol Oncol 1989;35(3):383–6.

[89] Rose PG. Skin bridge recurrences in vulvar cancer: frequency and management. Int J Gynecol Cancer 1999;9(6):508–11.

[90] Hacker N. Vulva cancer. In: Berek J, Hacker N, editors. Practical gynecologic oncology. Baltimore: Williams and Wilkins; 1989. p. 391–423.

[91] De Hullu JA, Hollema H, Lolkema S, et al. Vulvar carcinoma. The price of less radical surgery. Cancer 2002;95(11):2331–8.

[92] De Hullu JA, Oonk MH, Van Der Zee AG. Modern management of vulvar cancer. Curr Opin Obstet Gynecol 2004;16(1):65–72.

[93] Geisler J, Manahan K, Buller R, et al. Neoadjuvant chemotherapy in vulvar cancer: avoiding primary exenteration. Presented at the 35th Annual Meeting of the Society of Gynecologic Oncology. San Diego, February 7–11, 2004.

[94] Levenback C, Burke TW, Gershenson DM, et al. Intraoperative lymphatic mapping for vulvar cancer. Obstet Gynecol 1994;84(2):163–7.

ELSEVIER
SAUNDERS

Surg Oncol Clin N Am
14 (2005) 633–648

SURGICAL
ONCOLOGY CLINICS
OF NORTH AMERICA

Radical Operations for Soft Tissue Sarcomas

John M. Kane III, MD, William G. Kraybill, MD*

*Department of Surgical Oncology–Melanoma/Sarcoma, Roswell Park Cancer Institute,
Elm and Carlton Streets, Buffalo, NY 14263, USA*
State University of New York at Buffalo, Buffalo, NY 14214, USA

The term "radical" has different meanings based upon the context in which it is used. From a purely medical standpoint, radical is defined as "directed to the cause; directed to the root or source of a morbid process, as radical surgery" [1]. However, in a more familiar sense, radical is often taken to mean "departing markedly from the usual or customary; extreme" [2]. In regard to the treatment of sarcomas, the former definition would apply to any treatment that was potentially curative in nature. In contrast, it is the latter definition that conjures up images of very extensive operations, major amputations, and unique methods of reconstruction. To appreciate the true meaning of radical surgery for sarcomas, one needs to view the treatment of this disease from an historic perspective as the definition of radical changes based upon the prevailing wisdom of a given time period. As the significant contributions to the treatment of sarcomas span nearly one and a half centuries, the purpose of this review is not to be definitive but to highlight selected topics that have redefined the "radical" therapeutic approaches to this disease.

The rise of "radical" amputation

The idea of a sarcoma as a distinct type of cancer was not formalized until the mid 1800s by Virchow [3]. At that time, there were no adjuvant therapies such as radiation or chemotherapy. In addition, the concept of the pseudocapsule with surrounding foci of malignant cells was not been fully

* Corresponding author. Department of Surgical Oncology, Roswell Park Cancer Institute, Elm and Carlton Streets, Buffalo, NY 14263.
E-mail address: william.kraybill@roswellpark.org (W.G. Kraybill).

1055-3207/05/$ - see front matter © 2005 Elsevier Inc. All rights reserved.
doi:10.1016/j.soc.2005.04.001 *surgonc.theclinics.com*

appreciated until the late 1950s [4]. As a consequence, local excision of sarcomas was associated with very high local recurrence rates of 30% to 93% [5–9]. In addition, it was also appreciated that many patients with soft tissue sarcomas died secondary to distant metastases. Similar to the classic Halstedian thinking for other cancers such as carcinoma of the breast, it was felt that a very extensive surgical resection of the primary tumor might prevent the progression to distant metastatic disease. "The impression is that recurrences represent a real hazard to the patient. More than 50% of the patients with recurrences also developed concurrent distant metastases, and the cures even after additional therapy were few" [10]. This eventually led to the consensus that amputation was the appropriate treatment for extremity sarcomas. For a particular tumor site, the optimal level of amputation was typically above the joint proximal to the tumor.

This concept spurred the development of very extensive amputations such as hemipelvectomy, forequarter amputation, and even translumbar resection. Given that little emphasis was placed upon reconstruction, many of these amputations were extremely "radical" for the patient in terms of both physical appearance and functionality. To quote Dr. Theodore Miller, "I seldom tell the patient more than 24 hours in advance that the amputation must be done. This avoids the usual scramble by the family and the patient for other options which are readily available from radiotherapists, chemotherapists, and others, which only delay the definitive treatment of a lethal tumor. The surgeon who practices amputation in the treatment of malignant tumors of soft somatic tissues will, in general, have a higher curer rate than the surgeon who allows sentiment to interfere with his judgment and ill advisedly practices muscle block excision or other compromise operations" [11].

Hemipelvectomy

The first successful hemipelvectomy was reported by Charles Girard, in 1895, for a recurrent osteosarcoma [12]. Over the next several decades, hemipelvectomy (also known as interpelvic, interilioabdominal, internominoabdominal, interiliosacropubic, transiliac, or hindquarter amputation) became the standard surgical treatment for sarcomas of the proximal lower extremity, inguinal region, buttock, and musculoskeletal hemipelvis. From a technical standpoint, the procedure is rather straightforward, and entails removal of the hemipelvis from the sacroiliac joint to the symphysis pubis with the ipsilateral lower extremity. Typically, the major vessels are transected at the iliac level with preservation of the ureter and intra-abdominal structures. Depending upon the location of the primary tumor, soft tissue coverage of the defect is usually derived from a posterior gluteal-based flap. However, anterior and medial flaps (with preservation of the femoral vessels) have been described for more posteriorly based tumors [13,14]. As stated by Pringle, in 1916, this procedure "entails the greatest mutilation for which surgery is responsible; the wound made is an extremely large one, and the effect on the vitality of the patient must always be extremely severe" [15]. A typical high-grade sarcoma of the proximal thigh requiring hemipelvectomy with a posteriorly based flap is depicted in Fig. 1.

In the early years of hemipelvectomy, the procedure was associated with very high mortality rates of approximately 20% to 60% [16,17]. More acceptable mortality rates for modern series are in the range of 0% to 9% [18–24]. However, complications still occur in 50% to 80% of patients, and include hemorrhage, wound infection, skin flap necrosis (often with a wedge-shaped central defect), urethral or bladder fistulae, postoperative anemia secondary to loss of the marrow volume, and occasional late phantom pain [11,18,19,24,25]. Despite the lack of a fascial closure, significant herniation is rare and usually a late event [21]. Although many patients learn to ambulate with crutches, the rate of prosthesis use is fairly low, at less than 20% [18,23,25]. For the small number of series with long-term outcome, overall survival is in the range of 12% to 86% [18–24].

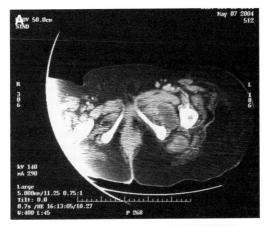

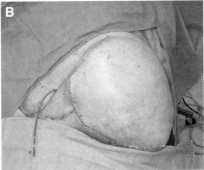

Fig. 1. A large high-grade sarcoma of the left medial thigh requiring formal hemipelvectomy. (*A*) CT scan showing the proximity of the tumor to the hemipelvis. (*B*) Primary closure with a posteriorly based flap.

Forequarter amputation

The first successful forequarter amputation was performed by Grosby, in 1836, for osteosarcoma. This technique (also known as interscapulothoracic or shoulder girdle amputation) has been used as the primary treatment for sarcomas of the proximal upper extremity, axilla with neurovascular involvement, and periscapular area. Subsequent modifications were employed to also include tumors invading the chest wall (radical transthoracic forequarter amputation) [26]. This procedure, with the resultant chest wall defect and subsequent reconstruction, is shown in Fig. 2. Anatomically, forequarter amputation entails division of the subclavian vessels and brachial plexus with removal of the upper extremity, scapula, and associated musculature. Both an anterior and posterior approach have been described. Reconstruction of the ensuing defect is typically with a deltoid-based flap. Compared with hemipelvectomy, the physiologic stress to the patients is minimal. Morbidity and mortality rates for this procedure have ranged from 0% to 5% and 0% to 24%, respectively [27,28]. Potential complications include wound infection, rare flap necrosis, and occasional phantom pain. Overall survival has been in the range of 25% to 80% [27,28].

Extended lower body amputations

Although sarcomas of the extremities are readily amenable to amputation, the treatment options for tumors involving portions of the lumbosacral region or even the entire pelvis are extremely limited. The technique of extended hemipelvectomy has been reported for tumors of the sacroiliac joint, and entails resection of portions of the lumbar spine, sacrum, and the

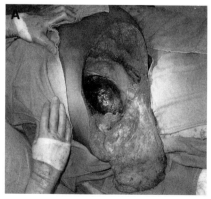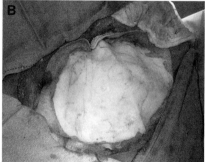

Fig. 2. Left forequarter amputation with en bloc chest wall resection for a recurrent high-grade sarcoma encasing the brachial plexus and the axillary vessels. (*A*) The surgical defect, including a major portion of the chest wall. (*B*) Reconstruction of the chest wall defect with polypropylene mesh and methyl methacrylate.

ilium. In a series of 18 patients with both bony and soft tissue sarcomas, the most common complication was wound-healing problems requiring extensive debridements and muscle flaps [29]. The local recurrence rate was only 15%, and 5-year overall survival was 72%.

Without challenge, the most radical of all potential sarcoma surgeries is the translumbar amputation or hemicorporectomy. First postulated by Kredel, in 1950 (as the "halfectomy"), but not successfully performed until 1961 by Aust and Absolon, this rare procedure has been reserved for extensive but isolated benign and malignant processes involving the pelvis, including skeletal and soft tissue tumors [30,31]. In essence, this operation entails amputation at the level of the lumbar spine with division of the spinal cord and resection of the bony pelvis, the rectum, the genitourinary structures, and both lower extremities. Due to the magnitude of the procedure, a two-stage approach is typically recommended [32,33]. The first stage entails laparotomy to ensure the potential resectability of the tumor. At this time, the GI and urinary diversions are created, with the stomas placed proximal to the umbilicus. At the second stage, the amputation and stump closure is performed. Previous stoma formation also reduces the chances of central nervous system contamination at the time of spinal cord transection and subsequent meningitis. Complications associated with this procedure include intraoperative hypotension following division of the cauda equina, an increased risk for postoperative pulmonary edema due to the loss of the third space capacity of the lower body, gastrointestinal or genitourinary fistulae, infectious complications such as meningitis, and significant wound-healing problems [33]. The latter occurs so frequently that prophylactic harvesting and banking of skin grafts from the lower extremities at the time of amputation is advocated. Rehabilitation consists of creation of a "bucket" prosthesis to maintain stability in an upright position.

The emphasis on limb salvage

Beginning as early as the 1930s, the necessity of amputation in all cases of soft tissue sarcoma began to be questioned. In 1958, Bowden and Booher published a classic paper on the fundamental shift in the principles and techniques of sarcoma surgery. "While in no sense intending to deprecate amputation as a means of treatment in certain situations, we herewith submit a method of surgical treatment which is consistent with the natural behavior of these tumors, which satisfies the tenets of good cancer surgery, and which obviates in selected instances the loss of an extremity" [34]. In a series of 36 patients treated with limb sparing muscle group wide excision, their local recurrence rate was a very reasonable 16%. A critical point at that time, which is often taken for granted in the era of routine preoperative imaging, was "the exact location and extent of a sarcoma cannot be determined by preoperative findings…it may be suggested that incisions were overly generous and that certain structures were unnecessarily sacrificed."

In 1975, Shiu and colleagues [35] reported on 297 patients with lower extremity sarcomas treated with either en bloc wide excision (n = 158) or amputation (n = 139) from 1949 to 1968. Although the two groups were not completely comparable, local recurrence and 5-year overall survival for wide excision versus amputation were 28% versus 7% and 63% versus 45%, respectively. There were also several important observations from this study that helped to reshape the approach to sarcoma surgery. First, the local recurrence rate for limb salvage in previously untreated patients was only 17%. Second, histologic tumor type, grade, and size were predictors of survival independent of the surgical therapy. Finally, local recurrence was not necessarily associated with a poor outcome, as greater than 30% of patients could be salvaged by additional surgery.

Throughout the 1970s, the dominance of surgical resection alone for sarcomas was gradually challenged by multimodality therapy to include radiation and even chemotherapy. In 1973, Suit and colleagues [36] described 57 potential amputation patients treated with radiation therapy either following limited excision alone with no residual tumor (n = 46) or obvious primary/recurrent tumor simply excised before or after radiation (n = 11). Local control was 87% for the entire group and 100% for distal extremity tumors. Metastasis-free survival was 58% and comparable to traditional surgical therapy. Importantly, a functional extremity was ultimately maintained in 60% of patients. In a more formal manner, Eilber and colleagues [37] performed a prospective trial of preoperative intra-arterial chemotherapy and radiation followed by radial en bloc tumor resection with 65 soft tissue sarcoma patients. Local recurrence was 3%, and only 6% required amputation (including for treatment-related complications). At a median follow-up of 22 months, overall disease-free survival was 65%.

These ideas did not mature into the modern concept of multimodality limb conservation until the 1980s. One of the seminal studies to solidify the potential equivalence of limb conservation to amputation was performed by Rosenberg and colleagues [38] at the National Cancer Institute from 1975 to 1981. In a prospective, randomized trial of patients with high-grade extremity sarcomas, 16 patients underwent amputation versus 27 patients treated with wide excision and adjuvant radiation. Although there was a slight difference in local recurrence for limb salvage versus amputation (15% versus 0%, $P = .06$), there was no difference in 5-year disease-free (71% versus 78%, $P = .75$) or overall survival (83% versus 88%, $P = .99$). Based upon the results from this and other studies, a National Institute of Health Consensus Development Conference in 1984 on "Limb-Sparing Treatment of Adult Soft Tissue Sarcomas" concluded that there is clearly a role for limb-sparing surgery, often by combining surgery with radiation or chemotherapy [39]. From this point forward, the emphasis on the treatment of soft tissue sarcomas shifted from extensive amputations to limb preservation strategies, postresection functionality, and quality of life.

Modern "radical" resection and reconstructive approaches

In essence, the new "radical" surgery for sarcomas has become complex reconstructions and limb salvage techniques. Major contributions to this treatment approach include microvascular plastic surgical techniques, an increased emphasis on functionality, the development of prosthetic materials, neurovascular reconstruction, downstaging with isolated limb perfusion, and the concept of limb remodeling and replantation.

Soft tissue coverage and reconstruction

Due to the greater emphasis on limb salvage, the need for adequate soft tissue coverage has increased dramatically. As opposed to amputation, wide excision often produces a very large surgical defect in locations such as the distal extremity that are not readily amenable to primary closure. In addition, the use of radiation therapy has been a "double edged sword." Although it is very effective at eradicating microscopic residual tumor, it also renders the entire treatment field functionally ischemic, which can significantly impair wound healing. In the setting of preoperative radiation with or without chemotherapy, postoperative wound healing complications can be as high as 37% [40]. Finally, exposure of the major neurovascular structures or the use of prosthetic reconstruction materials requires well-vascularized soft tissue coverage.

Frequently used pedicled local flaps (either as muscle alone or a myocutaneous unit) include the latissimus dorsi, pectoralis major, radial forearm, rectus abdominus, gluteus, rectus femoris, sartorius, tensor fasciae lata, gracilis, gastrocnemius, and soleus [41]. An example of a pedicled rectus abdominus myocutaneous flap for reconstruction of a wide excision defect following neoadjuvant chemoradiation for a large high-grade sarcoma of the right anterior thigh is depicted in Fig. 3. Although these flaps may be adequate for some defects, their use can potentially add to local functional morbidity and also increases the treatment field size if adjuvant radiation therapy is necessary. Consequently, one of the greatest contributions to sarcoma limb salvage has been free tissue transfer with microvascular anastomosis that can provide well-vascularized soft tissue and skin coverage for almost any part of the body. Commonly used free flaps include the transverse rectus abdominus myocutaneous, latissimus dorsi, radial forearm, and fibular or iliac crest osteocutaneous grafts when a portion of bone is needed for reconstruction [41]. Reported free flap survival even following adjuvant radiation therapy is a robust 75% to 100% [42,43].

Radical conceptual approaches to free flap reconstruction worth mentioning are the harvesting of the donor tissue from a planned amputation and free

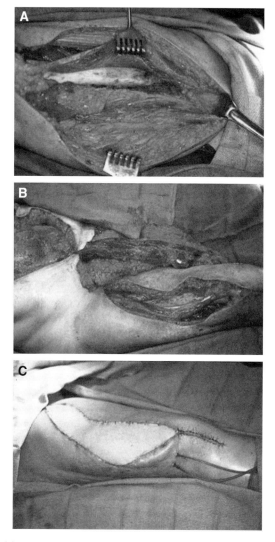

Fig. 3. Wide excision and reconstruction following neoadjuvant chemoradiation for a large high-grade sarcoma of the right anterior thigh. (*A*) The surgical defect, including exposed femur. (*B*) A pedicled ipsilateral rectus abdominus myocutaneous flap before placement in the surgical defect. (*C*) The formal wound closure with the pedicled flap.

muscle transfer with reinnervation to provide functional muscular contraction. As forequarter amputation frequently entails extensive soft tissue and even chest wall resection, a technique of total volar forearm musculocutaneous free flap harvest has been described for use in the soft tissue reconstruction [44]. The flap contains the entire musculature of the volar forearm with the overlying fascia and skin and is based upon a fairly long vascular pedicle consisting of the brachial artery and associated veins. A major benefit is the lack of donor-site morbidity as the tissue comes from the amputation specimen.

Although wide excision of a soft tissue sarcoma may allow for limb preservation, extensive muscular resection can result in significant functional disability. Therefore, an interesting alternative to simple replacement of soft tissue bulk is direct free muscle transfer with reinnervation. In a report by Doi and colleagues [45], this approach was employed in 17 patients with extremity soft tissue sarcomas undergoing major muscle group resection. Donor muscles included the latissimus dorsi, gracilis, rectus femoris, and tensor fasciae lata. The muscles were secured to bone proximally and tendon distally along with vascular and nerve anastomoses. Functional reconstructions included knee extension, knee flexion, toe/ankle extension, hip adduction, finger/wrist extension, and shoulder abduction. Muscle viability was 100% and reinnervation was successful in 94%. At a mean follow-up of 61 months, there were no local recurrences and the functional rating (using the Musculoskeletal Tumor Society scoring system) was very good at 87% for the lower extremity and 93% for the upper extremity.

Limb functionality and prosthetic reconstruction

The second most important contribution to limb salvage and functionality for sarcomas has been the development of prosthetic joints and allograft materials. Given that both the femur and the humerus have complex articulations proximally and distally, various combinations of arthrodesis, prosthetic implant, osteoarticular allograft, or allograft/implant have been employed. Although a detailed discussion of these options is beyond the scope of this review, their availability has increased the emphasis on functionality (even in the absence of joint reconstruction). The subsequent evolution of the hemipelvectomy and the forequarter amputation in light of these options deserve at least a brief mention.

In 1960, Sherman and Duthie [46] described the "conservative hemipelvectomy" as a modification more radical than hip disarticulation but more conservative than standard hemipelvectomy. Also known as a partial pelvectomy or conservative hemipelvectomy, the essential difference is that the sacroiliac joint and various portions of the ilium are preserved by bone division at or near the sciatic notch [47]. The principle advantages of this approach are its simplicity and preservation of the iliac crest for improved balance and prosthesis fitting [47,48]. The natural evolution of this technique was the development of the limb-sparing "internal hemipelvectomy" first described in the 1970s [49–51]. Internal hemipelvectomy entails resection of a portion of the hemipelvis with preservation of the lower extremity and allograft or prosthetic joint reconstruction. Complication rates (15–60%) and operative mortality (0–9%) are similar to that of traditional hemipelvectomy [52–56]. Reconstruction problems such as loosening or dislocation occur in 21% to 72% of patients but only 6% to 14% require conversion to amputation [53,55]. The ability to ambulate with minimal or no support is maintained in 93% to 100% of patients [52,54,56].

In contrast to the lower extremity, stable reconstruction at the level of the shoulder is not as critical given that the arm is not required for weight bearing or ambulation. However, even the best artificial limb is a very poor substitute for a functioning hand. As a consequence, limited resection of the scapulohumeral region is a potential option for preservation of a "normal" hand and lower arm. This approach was first reported by Linberg, in 1928, as the interscapulothoracic resection (Tikhoff-Linberg procedure), and consists of removal of the scapula, proximal humerus, and distal clavicle, with preservation of the vessels and brachial plexus [57]. Subsequent modifications include combinations of partial or complete resection of these bony structures with or without reconstruction of the joint. In the absence of arm stabilization by the humerus, the degree of flexion contracture at the elbow and a limited ability to elevate the hand are inversely associated with the length of the residual humeral stump [58]. These deficits are minimized with prosthetic or allograft stabilization/reconstruction [58,59]. Complications (such as infection, prosthetic instability, or late fracture) occur in 15% to 25% of patients, and are related more to the type of reconstruction as opposed to the resection itself [60]. Even in the absence of reconstruction, paresthesias and neuralgia are rare [58,59].

Treatment of major neurovascular involvement

Even in the era of limb salvage, involvement of the major neurovascular structures by tumor is frequently still considered an indication for amputation. Early experience with arterial and venous ligation without reconstruction often did not result in extremity ischemia, but produced significant edema [61]. With the development of reliable vascular conduits (saphenous vein grafts and prosthetic materials such as Dacron and Goretex), the possibility of vascular resection with reconstruction has been explored. Reported reconstructed arterial segments for sarcoma resection include iliac, femoral, popliteal, radial, and subclavian vessels [61–64]. There is still some debate regarding the need for venous reconstruction, with some authors advocating ligation while others recommend replacement (and even creation of an arteriovenous fistula to maintain venous patency). Arterial patency rates range from 92% to 100%, and local recurrence rates have been acceptable at 14% to 29% (especially given that resections are often performed for previously recurrent tumors) [61–64]. Wound infections and significant extremity edema occur infrequently. Important technical considerations include obtaining well-perfused soft tissue coverage of the vascular grafts and intraoperative manipulation of a joint traversed by a vascular conduit to identify potential kinking with postoperative movement [63,64].

Similar to the vessels, major nerve involvement by tumor has traditionally required amputation. For the upper extremity, sacrifice of the brachial plexus results in a functionless "bioprosthesis." Although loss of the femoral nerve in the lower extremity can be compensated for by a knee brace, it was previously felt that the morbidity associated with resection of the sciatic nerve was prohibitive. That tenet has been challenged based upon the functional results of several studies. Brooks and colleagues [65] examined the outcome of 18 patients undergoing sacrifice of the sciatic, tibial, or peroneal nerve at the time of sarcoma resection. Five patients experienced a local recurrence, but amputation was necessary in only one. Disease-free survival was 48% at 2 years. In the 11 surviving patients, 45% required an ankle brace for ambulation, but walking ability and distance was either unchanged or improved in 91%. Subjective postoperative functionality and quality of life were very good, and all patients preferred their limb salvage status over the prospects of amputation. In a similar study, Melendez and colleagues [66] investigated sciatic nerve reconstruction in six sarcoma patients. Five patients received autograft nerve reconstruction with either sural or peroneal nerves, and one underwent primary neurorrhaphy. There was partial distal sensation in 80% of the autografts, and the primary neurorrhaphy patient had some degree of both motor and sensory innervation. All surviving patients were ambulatory at the time of last follow-up. The authors concluded that motor and sensory reeducation with aggressive rehabilitation, even beginning preoperatively, can maximize the results of nerve grafting.

Isolated limb perfusion for locally advanced extremity sarcomas

Despite the advances in multimodality therapy and reconstructive techniques, a small proportion of patients with either a primary or recurrent extremity sarcoma will still require amputation for negative margin resection. Extrapolating from the results of isolated limb perfusion (ILP) for extremity in transit melanoma, this treatment approach has been examined as a potential limb-salvage modality for advanced extremity sarcomas. The largest experience comes from 186 patients perfused with melphalan and tumor necrosis factor (TNF) at eight centers across Europe (57% primary and 43% recurrent) [67]. Criteria for ILP included multifocal primary tumors or multiply recurrent tumors within the extremity, solitary tumors with involvement of the neurovascular bundles or bone, and recurrent tumors in previously irradiated fields with no possibility for radical resection. Patients were treated with a 90-minute ILP consisting of TNF (3–4 mg), melphalan (10–13 mg/L of extremity volume), and 39 to 40°C hyperthermia with planned marginal resection of the tumor remnants 4 to 24 weeks after ILP. There was a 29% combined clinical and histologic response complete response rate and a 53% partial response rate. At a median follow-up of 22 months, the limb salvage rate was 82%. In the patients without synchronous metastases (n = 161), the disease-free and overall survival rates were 64% and 73%, respectively. Other studies using melphalan/TNF or doxorubicin with or without TNF have shown similar limb salvage rates of 85% to 92% [68,69].

Limb modification and replantation

For the lower extremity, stump length inversely correlates with the amount of energy expended to ambulate with a prosthesis. As a consequence, hip disarticulation even with a good prosthesis often results in markedly limited postoperative ambulation. Although large tumors of the posteromedial thigh would typically dictate amputation at the hip, a modified amputation of the distal thigh with removal of the abductor and hamstring muscle groups has been described as an option to preserve stump length [70]. With this approach, the femur and quadriceps can be amputated near the knee while the portion of the thigh containing the tumor is resected near the pelvis. The ultimate result is equivalent to an above-knee amputation. A similar concept is augmentation of an amputation stump with either an allograft or an autografts from the surgical specimen. In a series of 10 patients who required lower extremity amputation for sarcoma, augmentation resulted in an average increase in stump length of 42%, including a functional transfemoral amputation as opposed to hip disarticulation in three patients [71]. Despite the use of an autograft in seven patients, local recurrence was rare at only 10%. An even more extreme approach described in the literature is conversion of a hip disarticulation to a functional above-knee amputation by replacement of the femur with a metallic hip prosthesis implanted into an inverted tibia and fibula [72].

Prosthetic limbs, even using space-age materials and design, are not comparable to a natural joint or extremity. In addition, the intricate function of the hand is almost impossible to reproduce. As a consequence, resection-replantation has occasionally been employed as an extreme form of limb sparing (as opposed to salvage). For the lower extremity, the rotationplasty was adapted from the treatment of congenital femur abnormalities for sarcomas of leg in the 1970s [73]. Conceptually, the modified Van Nes rotationplasty converts an above-knee amputation to an almost below-knee amputation with a functional knee-like joint. As described by Krajbich, the procedure entails resection of the thigh and knee with preservation of the sciatic nerve to the remaining distal leg and foot [74]. Following resection of the tumor, the distal stump is rotated 180 degrees and the tibia is fixed to the proximal femur. Vascular reanastomosis is performed, if necessary. This produces a posteriorly facing foot with the ankle joint positioned to serve as a "knee." The distal foot is then used for placement of a "below-knee" prosthesis. Potential advantages include a low complication rate and a greater ability to ultimately minimize leg length discrepancy in skeletally immature children. Functionality and quality of life also appear to be better compared with amputation [75].

A similar approach in the upper extremity has been used to maintain a functioning hand for tumors that may otherwise require forequarter amputation. First described by Windhager and colleagues [76], resection-replantation of the arm entails resecting a segment of the upper arm including bone, soft tissues, and even neurovascular structures. The distal arm is then replanted with vascular and neural reconstructions, if necessary. In a series of 12 patients, the complication rate was 33%, and one patient required secondary amputation due to pain. There were no local recurrences, but 50% of patients succumbed to distant metastatic disease. Fifty-eight percent of patients had "good to excellent" functional outcome and hand function was unrestricted in the six patients who did not undergo resection of the nerves.

Summary

Before the concept of multimodality therapy, the only expectation of surgical resection for the treatment of cancer was to obtain control of locoregional disease and hopefully prevent distant metastases. As a consequence, "radical" had a very precise definition, as it described the magnitude of the operation necessary to obtain negative margins. This philosophy led to the development of many "classic" procedures such as the radical mastectomy for breast cancer, abdominoperineal resection for rectal cancer, and major amputations for soft tissue sarcomas. For sarcoma patients, loss of functionality was the "price paid" for the treatment of their tumors. In the modern era of cancer treatment, "radical" is now a more abstract term that refers to a fundamental shift in our paradigms on cancer biology and the outcome of the patient, both oncologic and functional. For soft tissue sarcomas, this has led to innovative and sometimes extreme approaches such as free tissue transfer, major prosthetic reconstruction, and even limb replanation for treating the tumor in the setting of maximal functionality. The ability of routine preoperative imaging to accurately predict the location of the tumor must also be recognized as a significant contribution to limb-conserving surgery. As a consequence, although amputation was once considered the standard of care for extremity sarcomas, "amputation-free survival" has become an important clinical outcome in the treatment of this disease.

References

[1] Dorland's Illustrated Medical Dictionary. Philadelphia: W.B. Saunders; 2002.
[2] The American Heritage Dictionary of the English Language. 4th edition. New York: Houghton Mifflin; 2000.

[3] Virchow R. Die krankhaften Geschwulste. Berlin: August Hirschwald; 1863–7.
[4] Bowden L, Booher R. The principles and technique of resection of soft parts for sarcoma. Surgery 1958;44:963–76.
[5] Cantin J, McNeer G, Chu F, et al. The problem of local recurrence after treatment of soft tissue sarcoma. Ann Surg 1968;168:47–53.
[6] Stout A. Fibrosarcoma—the malignant tumor of fibroblasts. Cancer 1948;1:30–59.
[7] Markhede G, Angervall L, Stener B. A multivariate analysis of the prognosis after surgical treatment of malignant soft tissue tumors. Cancer 1982;49:1721–33.
[8] Gerner R, Moore G, Pickren J. Soft tissue sarcomas. Ann Surg 1985;31:803–8.
[9] Rosenberg S, Glatstein E. Perspectives on the role of surgery and radiation therapy in the treatment of soft tissue sarcoma of the extremities. Semin Oncol 1981;8: 190–200.
[10] Brennhovd I. The treatment of soft tissue sarcomas—a plea for a more urgent and aggressive approach. Acta Chir Scand 1966;131:438–42.
[11] Miller T. 100 cases of hemipelvectomy: a personal experience. Surg Clin North Am 1974;54: 905–13.
[12] Girard C. IX Congress Franc De Chir., 1894;12:585–96.
[13] Frey C, Mathews L, Benjamin H, et al. A new technique for hemipelvectomy. Surg Gynecol Obstet 1976;143:753–6.
[14] Luna-Perez P, Herrera L. Medial thigh myocutaneous flap for covering extended hemi-pelvectomy. Eur J Surg Oncol 1995;21:623–6.
[15] Pringle J. The interpelvic-abdominal amputation. Br J Surg 1916;4:283–96.
[16] King D, Steelquist J. Transiliac amputation. J Bone Joint Surg 1943;25:351.
[17] Beck N, Bickel W. Internominoabdominal amputation. J Bone Joint Surg 1948;30A:201–9.
[18] Butzelaar R, Fortner J. Results of hemipelvectomy for soft tissue sarcoma. Neth J Surg 1981; 33:79–82.
[19] Pack G, Miller T. Exarticulation of the innominate bone and corresponding lower extremity (hemipelvectomy) for primary and metastatic cancer. A report of one hundred and one cases with analysis of the end results. J Bone Joint Surg Am 1964;46:91–5.
[20] Funk F, Jernigan S. Sarcomas of the pelvis: hemipelvectomy. J Med Assoc Ga 1957;46: 333–5.
[21] Miller T. Hemipelvectomy in lower extremity tumors. Orthop Clin North Am 1977;8: 903–19.
[22] Baliski C, Schachar N, McKinnon J, et al. Hemipelvectomy: a changing perspective for a rare procedure. Can J Surg 2004;47:99–103.
[23] Carter S, Eastwood D, Grimer R, et al. Hindquarter amputation for tumours of the musculoskeletal system. J Bone Joint Surg Br 1990;72:490–3.
[24] Prewitt T, Alexander H, Sindelar W. Hemipelvectomy for soft tissue sarcoma: clinical results in fifty-three patients. Surg Oncol 1995;4:261–9.
[25] Douglass H, Razack M, Holyoke E. Hemipelvectomy. Arch Surg 1975;110:82–5.
[26] Stafford E, Williams G. Radical transthoracic forequarter amputation. Ann Surg 1958;148: 699.
[27] Fanous N, Didolkar M, Holyoke E, et al. Evaluation of forequarter amputation in malignant diseases. Surg Gynecol Obstet 1976;142:381–4.
[28] Ham S, Hoekstra H, Schraffordt Koops H, et al. The interscapulothoracic amputation in the treatment of malignant diseases of the upper extremity with a review of the literature. Eur J Surg Oncol 1993;19:543–8.
[29] Fuchs B, Yaszemski M, Sim F. Combined posterior pelvis and lumbar spine resection for sarcoma. Clin Orthop 2002;397:12–8.
[30] Ferrara B. Hemicorporectomy: the contribution of Frederick E. Kredel. J S C Med Assoc 1988;84:83–4.
[31] Aust J, Absolon K. A successful lumbosacral amputation, hemicorporectomy. Surgery 1960; 48:756–9.

[32] Miller T, Mackenzie A, Randall H. Translumbar amputation for advanced cancer: indications and physiologic alterations in four cases. Ann Surg 1966;164:514–21.
[33] Weaver J, Flynn M. Hemicorporectomy. J Surg Oncol 2000;73:117–24.
[34] Bowden L, Booher R. The principles and technique of resection of soft parts for sarcoma. 1958. Clin Orthop 2004;426:5–10.
[35] Shiu M, Castro E, Hajdu S, et al. Surgical treatment of 297 soft tissue sarcomas of the lower extremity. Ann Surg 1975;182:597–602.
[36] Suit H, Russell W, Martin R. Management of patients with sarcoma of soft tissue in an extremity. Cancer 1973;31:1247–55.
[37] Eilber F, Mirra J, Grant T, et al. Is amputation necessary for sarcomas? A seven-year experience with limb salvage. Ann Surg 1980;192:431–8.
[38] Rosenberg SA, Tepper J, Glatstein E, et al. The treatment of soft-tissue sarcomas of the extremities: prospective randomized evaluations of (1) limb-sparing surgery plus radiation therapy compared with amputation and (2) the role of adjuvant chemotherapy. Ann Surg 1982;196:305–15.
[39] Consensus Conference. Limb-sparing treatment of adult soft-tissue sarcomas and osteosarcomas. JAMA 1985;254:1791–4.
[40] Bujko K, Suit H, Springfield D, et al. Wound healing after preoperative radiation for sarcoma of soft tissues. Surg Gynecol Obstet 1993;176:124–34.
[41] Langstein H, Robb G. Reconstructive approaches in soft tissue sarcoma. Semin Surg Oncol 1999;17:52–65.
[42] Heiner J, Rao V, Mott W. Immediate free tissue transfer for distal musculoskeletal neoplasms. Ann Plast Surg 1993;30:140–6.
[43] Krag D, Klein H, Schneider P, et al. Composite tissue transfer in limb-salvage surgery. Arch Surg 1991;126:639–41.
[44] Cordeiro P, Cohen S, Burt M, et al. The total volar forearm musculocutaneous free flap for reconstruction of extended forequarter amputations. Ann Plast Surg 1998;40:388–96.
[45] Doi K, Kuwata N, Kawakami F, et al. Limb-sparing surgery with reinnervated free-muscle transfer following radical excision of soft-tissue sarcoma in the extremity. Plast Reconstr Surg 1999;104:1679–87.
[46] Sherman C, Duthie R. Modified hemipelvectomy. Cancer 1960;13:51.
[47] Rush B, Brower T. Partial pelvectomy for sarcomas of the lower extremity. South Med J 1969;62:319–22.
[48] Ariel I, Shah J. The conservative hemipelvectomy. Surg Gynecol Obstet 1977;144:406–13.
[49] Steel H. Partial or complete resection of the hemipelvis. J Bone Joint Surg Am 1978;60:719–30.
[50] Burri C, Claes L, Gerngross H, et al. Total "internal" hemipelvectomy. Arch Orthop Trauma Surg 1979;94:219–26.
[51] Eilber F, Grant T, Sakai D, et al. Internal hemipelvectomy-excision of the hemipelvis with limb preservation. An alternative to hemipelvectomy. Cancer 1979;43:806–9.
[52] Apffelstaedt J, Driscoll DL, Karakousis CP. Partial and complete internal hemipelvectomy: complications and long-term follow-up. J Am Coll Surg 1995;181:43–8.
[53] Ham S, Schraffordt Koops H, Veth R, et al. External and internal hemipelvectomy for sarcomas of the pelvic girdle: consequences of limb-salvage treatment. Eur J Surg Oncol 1997;23:540–6.
[54] Lewis S, Wunder J, Couture J, et al. Soft tissue sarcomas involving the pelvis. J Surg Oncol 2001;77:8–14.
[55] Wirbel R, Schulte M, Mutschler W. Surgical treatment of pelvic sarcomas: oncologic and functional outcome. Clin Orthop 2001;390:190–205.
[56] Kollender Y, Shabat S, Bickels J, et al. Internal hemipelvectomy for bone sarcomas in children and young adults: surgical considerations. Eur J Surg Oncol 2000;26:398–404.
[57] Linberg B. Interscapulo-thoracic resection for malignant tumors of the shoulder joint region. J Bone Joint Surg 1928;26:344–9.

[58] Kotz R, Salzer M. Resection therapy of malignant tumours of the shoulder girdle. Osterr Kneipp Mag 1975;2:97–109.

[59] Ham S, Hoekstra H, Eisma W, et al. The Tikhoff-Linberg procedure in the treatment of sarcomas of the shoulder girdle. J Surg Oncol 1993;53:71–7.

[60] Kneisl JS. Function after amputation, arthrodesis, or arthroplasty for tumors about the shoulder. J South Orthop Assoc 1995;4:228–36.

[61] Fortner J, Kim D, Shiu M. Limb-preserving vascular surgery for malignant tumors of the lower extremity. Arch Surg 1977;112:391–4.

[62] Karakousis C, Karmpaliotis C, Driscoll D. Major vessel resection during limb-preserving surgery for soft tissue sarcomas. World J Surg 1996;20:345–9.

[63] Imparato A, Roses D, Francis K, et al. Major vascular reconstruction for limb salvage in patients with soft tissue and skeletal sarcomas of the extremities. Surg Gynecol Obstet 1978; 147:891–6.

[64] Steed D, Peitzman A, Webster M, et al. Limb sparing operations for sarcomas of the extremities involving critical arterial circulation. Surg Gynecol Obstet 1987;164:493–8.

[65] Brooks A, Gold J, Graham D, et al. Resection of the sciatic, peroneal, or tibial nerves: assessment of functional status. Ann Surg Oncol 2002;9:41–7.

[66] Melendez M, Brandt K, Evans G. Sciatic nerve reconstruction: limb preservation after sarcoma resection. Ann Plast Surg 2001;46:375–81.

[67] Eggermont A, Schraffordt Koops H, Klausner J, et al. Isolated limb perfusion with tumor necrosis factor and melphalan for limb salvage in 186 patients with locally advanced soft tissue extremity sarcomas. The cumulative multicenter European experience. Ann Surg 1996; 224:756–64.

[68] Gutman M, Inbar M, Lev-Shlush D, et al. High dose tumor necrosis factor-alpha and melphalan administered via isolated limb perfusion for advanced limb soft tissue sarcoma results in a >90% response rate and limb preservation. Cancer 1997;79:1129–37.

[69] Rossi C, Foletto M, Di Filippo F, et al. Soft tissue limb sarcomas: Italian clinical trials with hyperthermic antiblastic perfusion. Cancer 1999;86:1742–9.

[70] Stener B. Amputation through the lower thigh with removal of the adductor and hamstring muscles. An alternative to hip joint disarticulation in certain cases of malignant soft-tissue tumor. Clin Orthop 1971;80:133–8.

[71] Mohler D, Kessler J, Earp B. Augmented amputations of the lower extremity. Clin Orthop 2000;371:183–97.

[72] Wieder H, Nicholson J. Total resection of femur with turn-up plasty of tibia and prosthetic replacement of hip joint. Ann Surg 1956;144:271–6.

[73] Kotz R, Salzer M. Rotation-plasty for childhood osteosarcoma of the distal part of the femur. J Bone Joint Surg 1982;64A:959.

[74] Krajbich J. Modified Van Nes rotationplasty in the treatment of malignant neoplasms in the lower extremities of children. Clin Orthop 1991;262:74–7.

[75] Hillmann A, Gosheger G, Hoffmann C, et al. Rotationplasty—surgical treatment modality after failed limb salvage procedure. Arch Orthop Trauma Surg 2000;120:555–8.

[76] Windhager R, Millesi H, Kotz R. Resection-replantation for primary malignant tumours of the arm. An alternative to fore-quarter amputation. J Bone Joint Surg Br 1995;77:176–84.

SURGICAL
ONCOLOGY CLINICS
OF NORTH AMERICA

ELSEVIER
SAUNDERS

Surg Oncol Clin N Am
14 (2005) 649–653

Index

Note: Page numbers of article titles are in **boldface** type.

Changing Your Address?

Make sure your subscription changes too! When you notify us of your new address, you can help make our job easier by including an exact copy of your Clinics label number with your old address (see illustration below.) This number identifies you to our computer system and will speed the processing of your address change. Please be sure this label number accompanies your old address and your corrected address—you can send an old Clinics label with your number on it or just copy it exactly and send it to the address listed below.

We appreciate your help in our attempt to give you continuous coverage. Thank you.

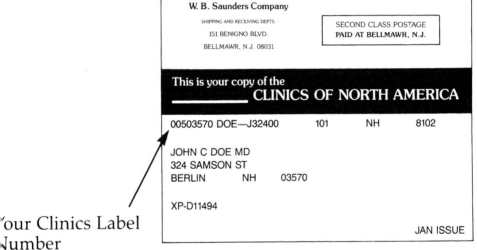

Your Clinics Label Number
Copy it exactly or send your label along with your address to:
W.B. Saunders Company, Customer Service
Orlando, FL 32887-4800
Call Toll Free 1-800-654-2452

Please allow four to six weeks for delivery of new subscriptions and for processing address changes.